Practical
Folk
Medicine
of Hawai'i

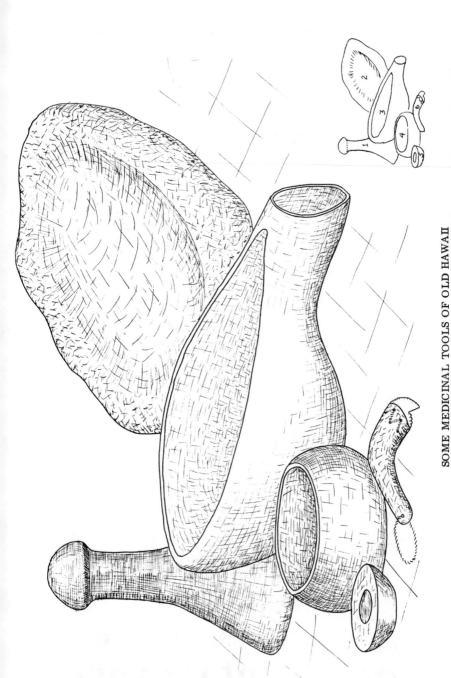

SOME MEDICINAL TOOLS OF OLD HAWAII

1. Stone Pounder 2. Stone Salt Pan 3. Gourd Strainer 4. Wood Bowl 5. Stone Kahuna Cup 6. Shark Tooth Knife

Practical
Folk Medicine
of
Hawai'i

Text & Illustrations
by
Likeke R. McBride

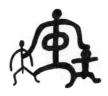

Dedicated to
Charlotte Armstrong Lewis

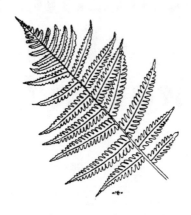

ISBN 0-912180-27-7
Library of Congress Catalog Card Number: 76-1272

Published in Hawai'i by the
Petroglyph Press, Ltd.
160 Kamehameha Avenue - Hilo, Hawai'i 96720
Phone (808) 935-6006 - Fax (808) 935-1553
E-Mail: reedbook@interpac.net
www.basicallybooks.com

Thirteenth Printing - June 1999

CONTENTS

Page

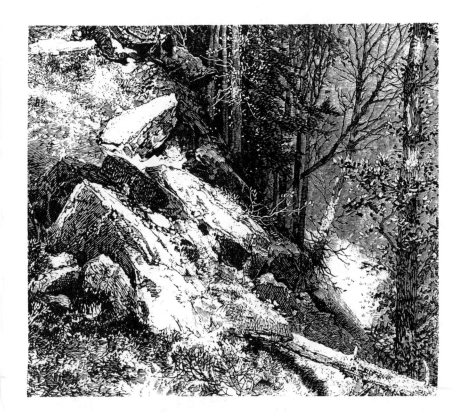

KILAUEA FOREST 1880

BEFORE YOU BEGIN

There is a scarcity of published information on Hawaii's folk medicine, and the little that is available is already out-of-date. Many of the medical recipes of the past are now almost useless because the plants called for no longer exist or are too difficult to find.

The creation of huge ranches and vast agricultural tracts, as well as urban spread, have decreased Hawaii's area of wild vegetation. Also harmful have been the depredations of introduced insect pests and feral animals, especially the goat. All of these have affected the native island plants, endangering some species and reducing the numbers of many more.

Selection of the remedies included in this book was made on the availability of plants, the ease of identifying them, and the simplicity of using them in folk medicine for common ailments.

It was not possible to include all of the remedies and their variations given to me. Contributors have sometimes disagreed on which treatment is best for a particular malady, and, just as often, have failed to concur on how some medicines are compounded. When there was too much disagreement, and the reason was not obvious, the treatment was left out of this book.

Sometimes several different recommendations have been included for the same condition. Principally, this is because some herbs are not available the year around. Also, different locations have widely divergent assemblages of plants. Individuals differ, too, and where one will be helped by a certain remedy, another will need one quite different.

As with all primitive peoples, home remedies most certainly have existed in Hawaii since ancient times. The earliest inhabitants of the islands undoubtedly learned which plants made well people sick and sick people well.

When the Polynesians arrived in Hawaii from distant lands a thousand years or more ago, they soon became the dominant group, setting up a caste system which relegated those people already living on the islands to a low rank. There was probably very little exchange of ideas. Instead of reliance on home medicine, there evolved a class of educated and trained professionals to head almost every endeavor. These were the *kahuna*. In the science of medicine they may have excelled or equaled the best physicians in the world of that time.

If anything was lacking in their medical repertoire it may have been preventive medicine. However, they did teach the importance of keeping fit. Contrary to popular belief, few Hawaiians of early times were overweight. The *kahunas* emphasized the importance of cleanliness to good health. Frequent bathing and internal cleansing were stressed. Illness required rest and restricted diet as well as medicine.

Kahunas deplored the use of folk medicine and exhorted the people to employ the services of *kahuna lapaʻau laʻau*. The poor and the isolated, however, continued to cling to their country ways. The ancient remedies lived on.

When the Europeans arrived they brought many plants which were new to the Hawaiians, among them onions, peppers, aloe and tobacco. The *kahuna lapaʻau laʻau* quickly learned the merits of some of these and adopted them for use in their remedies.

In 1819, four decades after Captain Cook discovered the islands, the Hawaiian "establishment" fell. The caste system was abolished and the professional classes disbanded, among them the physicians. The diseases brought by the foreigners, plus the lack of local doctors, caused the population to be reduced to less than half in a few years.

Folk medicine in Hawaii today consists of the remnants of the original home remedies, fragments of the knowledge of the *kahuna lapaʻau laʻau* and treatments that have come in with people from various places in the world.

The number of Hawaiians who have fundamental knowledge of the ancient medical practices is dwindling every day. Some of these people carry to their graves invaluable data concerning old remedies, because the secrets were under *kapu*. Thus, a great deal of information has already been lost.

Unfortunately, there is no one in Hawaii today that has all of the medical knowledge and skill of the *kahuna lapaʻau*. About 150 years have elapsed since the last of these received their formal training. The medical *kahuna* of old Hawaii began his education at an early age and studied plants and their effects intensively for 15 to 20 years. Not only did he have to learn the uses of over 300 plants, but the medical applications of materials taken from the ocean as well. In the last few years, extracts from certain species of marine life have been examined for use in treating cancer. The results have been favorable enough to warrant research into other old Hawaiian medical recipes which call for ingredients from the ocean. Perhaps from these endeavors will come solutions to medical problems that beset mankind. This would not surprise those old people today who remember the ancient Hawaiian prophecy, "From the sea shall come the life of the land."

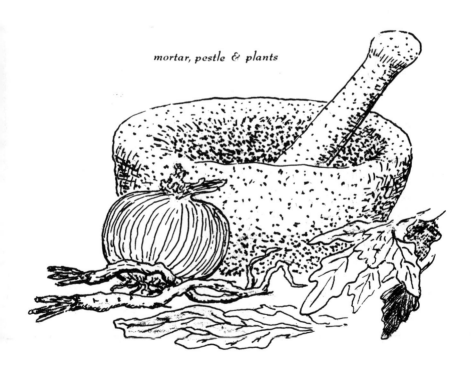

mortar, pestle & plants

AUTHOR'S ACKNOWLEDGEMENTS

I would like to record here my sincere *mahalo* to all of the island people who have helped me with this book. In a sense it is theirs, because without the assistance of the *kama'aina* it could never have been produced.

From my grandparents in the hills of Southeastern Ohio I learned the value of herbs in dealing with many common health problems. Not very strange, perhaps, is the fact that many of the practices of herbal medicine employed by the eastern Indians and country people of long ago are similar to those used by the Hawaiians. Thus, during World War II, when I first met Hawaiians, I felt a bond of sorts with the people who were so friendly and knew so much about folk medicine.

Some of the recipes in this book come from that time, taken from yellowed pages of notes with rusty staples. Others have been gathered during the past 14 years on the Island of Hawai'i. So many people have contributed suggestions and formulae that it is impossible to give individual credit. All of the assistance has been valuable, for even if not the first recommendation, it may have served to confirm the original.

Many of my informants through the years are no longer living. In spite of this, the recipes they shared but didn't want printed have been left out. Some of the "miracle" cures that I have been told of have also been omitted, not because I do not believe them, but for the reason that, in my opinion, they demonstrate a greater power than that of folk medicine.

Not only the Hawaiians but island people of various ethnic backgrounds have aided with the preparation of this book. To those who helped a little and to those who helped a lot, *mahalo nui loa.*

L. R. McBride
Volcano, Hawai'i
1975

WORDS OF WARNING

Since the treatments mentioned in this book grew out of the traditional folk medicine of the Hawaiian people, and have not been scientifically tested in most cases, neither the author nor the publisher endorses or makes any claim as to the efficacy, nor accepts any responsibility for their use. We strongly advise that in any serious condition your doctor be consulted before you begin the use of a home remedy.

Much of modern medicine, however, throughout the world is derived from plants, and in using and confirming the knowledge developed by the Hawaiians over many centuries, we are contributing to this process. The author believes that, within limitations, an individual should be able to choose the kind of medication he desires for any ailment which does not endanger others.

None of the medicines described in this book are recommended for children. Keep all medicines and medicinal plants away from children. Warn children of the danger of putting plant substances in their mouths.

Some of the plants mentioned in this book are listed as poisonous or potentially dangerous. The degree of toxicity of a number of these, such as *popolo*, has been highly controversial for many years. In most cases, the herbs and plants that might be considered unwise to take internally have been retained for use in external application only. Additional specific cautionary remarks concerning some plants are included in the recipes using them.

Do not eat a part of any plant or drink the juice of any plant that you do not know. There are some plants growing in Hawai'i that may cause sickness and death. For treatments which involve ingesting plants, it is wise to begin slowly to determine your personal tolerance to them.

Never treat two ailments at the same time. Doing so might involve bringing together plant materials which could interact unfavorably. The result might be the negation of one or both treatments or an undesirable side effect.

A correct diagnosis is the important part of medicinal practice. Dealing with a cut is generally a straightforward proposition. It is only necessary to stop the bleeding and prevent infection while the wound heals. Illness, however, is often a complex thing. It must be born in mind that one illness can simulate another. For example, treating a stomach-ache that is in reality appendicitis could be fatal.

Some readers may question the inclusion of turtle oil among the recipes since these animals may be endangered. The success of turtle farms in the Caribbean and new ones begun in the Pacific may soon turn this around and the qualities of turtle oil are too remarkable to let them be forgotten.

When gathering medicinal plants try to collect those that are less likely to be contaminated by agricultural plant sprays and automobile exhausts. Leave the isolated plant to multiply and take specimens from a place of abundance. While most plants mentioned in this book are fairly common, others such as *puakala* and some of the ferns seem to diminish in number every year. A sensible approach to obtaining these plants will insure that they will not become endangered.

The author does not claim to have tested or taken every remedy in this book. Undoubtedly, no one person has ever done so. Those that I have tried and that have been successful for me are included in this text.

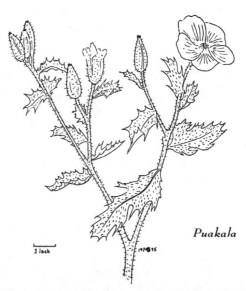

Puakala

1 inch

TOOLS AND TECHNIQUES

About a third of the plants used in Hawaii for medicine must be dug up to obtain the root. Since the ground conditions vary widely in the islands, a selection of digging implements will be helpful to have on hand.

One of the most useful tools is the o'o, developed by the ancient Hawaiians. Formerly it was made entirely of hard wood, but today the o'o consists of a wooden handle with the business end made of steel. The blade is about 3½ inches wide with a square tip and sloping shoulders. The socket fits a straight handle about the length of a long shovel. The kama'aina will tell you that the o'o is unexcelled for forest or woodland digging.

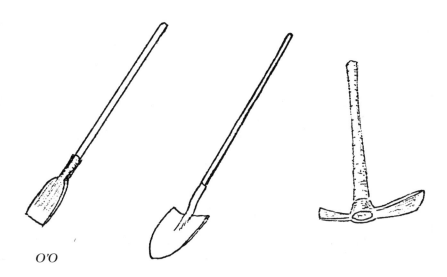

O'O

Large jobs such as unearthing huge *awa* roots will require the service of a mattock and a long handled shovel as well as the *o'o*.

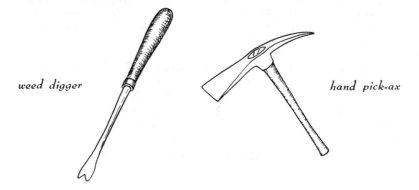

weed digger   *hand pick-ax*

Smaller roots can be extracted by using a weed digger or a hand pick-ax.

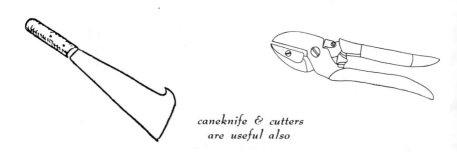

*caneknife & cutters
are useful also*

When digging roots make very sure that the root removed goes with the plant you have identified. Broken-off roots are best discarded unless you can be certain that they do belong to the stock being extracted. Put a tag on the fresh dug root and place it in an individual plastic bag. Label or tag the bag as well to prevent a mix-up. Work with only one root at a time during the washing and taking off of the outside bark.

The bark may be removed from roots by slitting the root on one side with a knife. Then, holding the knife by the blade, tap the root with the handle all over. This helps to loosen the bark. Next, start the removal at the larger end of the root by using the thumb nails, peeling off the bark with care. In most cases the bark can be most easily removed from the root while it is fresh.

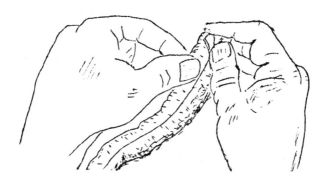

A sharp knife is a necessary part of the tool kit of the medicine maker. The most useful is an oilcloth or carpet knife with a blade that folds into the handle, thus enabling it to be safely carried in the pocket. This instrument is equally good for cutting plants and removing bark, although a small chisel is very helpful for the latter.

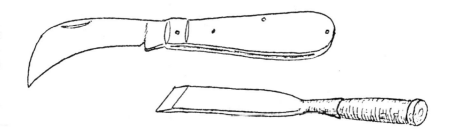

Remember, when taking a section of bark from a tree, cut it away only on one side. Removing the bark from entirely around the trunk will kill the tree as surely as cutting it down. Wet the piece of bark you have taken off with a little water before putting it in a plastic bag. This will make it easier to work with later.

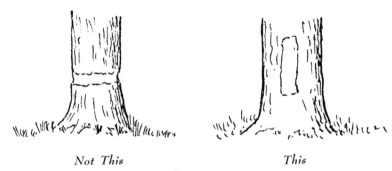

Not This   *This*

When gathering leaves, take a few from each plant around you rather than stripping one specimen. The old Hawaiians claimed that this practice insured a better medicine without harming any of the plants. Bag and label the leaves promptly to avoid future confusion.

Few things are as useful as plastic bags in gathering the materials for making medicine. They keep vegetative material from drying out and add almost no extra weight to be carried into the field. Just as important, they can be closed and labeled easily.

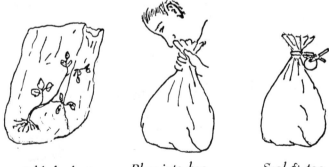

bag sprinkled plant   *Blow into bag*   *Seal & tag*

Many recipes require the ingredients to be crushed in order to extract the plant juices. Salt is added as a "getter" to facilitate this process. You can still use a stone and a pounding board just as the people have done from time immemorial to accomplish this, but it is time consuming and hard work. An ordinary food grinder will do much the same thing and save a great deal of labor. Grind the plant materials as suggested in the recipe, mixing the Hawaiian salt with the drier ingredients. Let the plants stand for a time in the brine before squeezing out the juice. At all stages of manufacture, remember to keep the medicine clean.

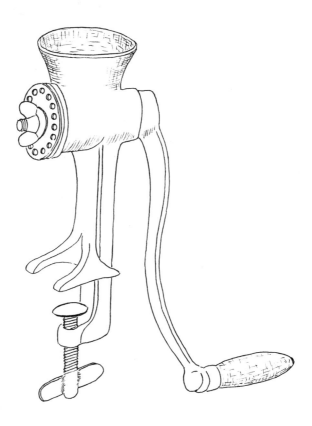

One of the more difficult phases of making folk medicine is that of squeezing out the juice from the crushed or ground material. Often this can be done by simply putting the pulp into a towel and twisting it. A handy trick is using a potato ricer first to get some of the juice out before resorting to the towel.

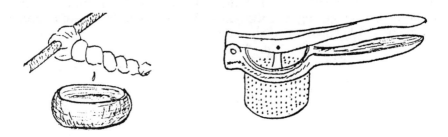

A more elaborate press can be made of a short length of three inch pipe and a "C" clamp. A disk of strong metal that just fits inside the pipe can be used for a piston head and a piece with many holes drilled in it can be the back-up plate.

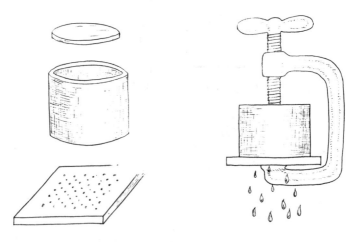

There are many ingenious arrangements that can be put together using the lever and fulcrum principle that will work as well as anything you can buy. Experiment a bit and find the method that operates best for you in extracting the fluid portion of the plants.

For small amounts a garlic press may be satisfactory, but regardless of how the juice is squeezed out it should be strained through cheese cloth or muslin to remove all of the fiber.

A pestle and mortar are hard to beat for grinding dry ingredients to powder. A set can be purchased at a scientific supply house or you may choose to make your own. Sometimes you can find a suitable stone at the beach that will do for the start of a mortar. Try to find one that is dense, with no *pukas* and a concave side. By pounding and grinding you can deepen it to something you can use . A long, rounded pebble of dense lava rock will make a fine pestle to complete a homemade set of tools that will probaably never wear out.

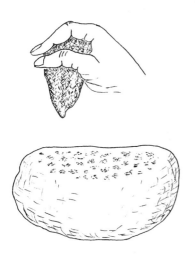

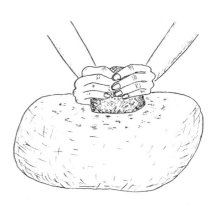

Peck with a dense rock　　　*Grind down with a rough rock*

WHERE IT'S AT

Given enough time and travel in remote places on most of the high islands of Hawaii, you would probably stumble across every plant mentioned in this text. To save time and effort, be observant! Read carefully the descriptions of the plants in this book. Each one is illustrated to emphasize the points of identification. About 60% of the described plants are very easy to obtain.

Whenever you happen to be in a new place notice the plant assemblages around you. A small notepad is helpful in recording where you find certain plants of medicinal value.

If you find an abundance, take home a couple of plants of each species. By simulating their natural surroundings you may be able to start a garden of wild herbs.

PLANTS THAT YOU CAN GROW

aloe	*awapuhi keokeo*	*ko'oko'olau*
awa	*kalo (taro)*	*lapine*
awapuhi	*ki (ti)*	

COMMON WEEDS

laukahi	*pohe kula*	*popolo*

THINGS YOU CAN BUY

aka'akai	Hawaiian salt	*pia* starch (arrowroot)
awapuhi pake	Hawaiian red salt	*'uala*

WHERE PLANTS CAN BE FOUND

UPLAND PLANTS—above 2000 feet altitude

a'ali'i	*ha'uoi*	*ohelo la'au*
amaumau	*ho'i'o*	*olapa*
hapu'u	*koa*	*pakikawaio*

LOWLAND PLANTS—below 2000 feet altitude

aloe	*iliohe*	*niu*
auhuhu	*iniko*	*noni*
awa	*ko*	*oliwa-ku-kahakai*
awapuhi	*ko'oko'olau*	*pia*
awapuhi pake	*kukui*	*pohe kula*
hau	*mikana*	*puakala*
ilie'e	*naupaka kahakai*	*uhaloa*
		ulu

UPLAND & LOWLAND PLANTS—up to 4000' feet altitude

'ape	*kuawa*	*pi'ipi'i-lau-manamana*
awapuhi keokeo	*limu kaha*	*pipi & moa*
ihi	*laukahi*	*popolo*
kalo	*ohia*	*pua-pilipili*
ki	*palepiwa*	*'ulei*
koali	*pepa*	

A'ALI'I

Dodonaea eriocarpa

A'ali'i is most frequently recognized as a shrub but may grow to a height of 25 feet or more. Generally, the two- to four-inch-long leaves are narrow with either a blunt or a pointed end. They are alternate with short stems and may be somewhat sticky at the branch tips. The most conspicuous characteristic is the cluster of red, reddish brown or brown papery seed capsules that adorn the plants. Each capsule is about one-half an inch long and has two to four "wings" or vanes. Hawaiians once used these to make a pink dye.

The a'ali'i can be found on all of the islands in the drier habitat ranging from 1,000 to 8,000 feet in altitude. It is most abundant at middle elevations between 2,500 to 6,000 feet.

The young leaves and branch tips are the portions of the plant that are gathered for medicine.

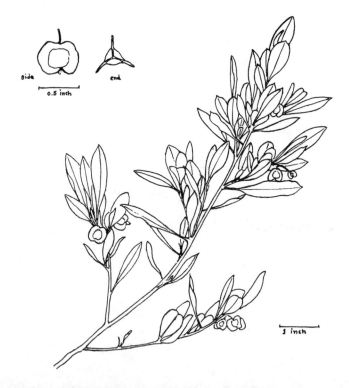

AKA'AKAI

Allum cepa

Aka'akai is the common onion. It obtained its name from the similarity of its tops to those of the great bullrush which grows on the edge of marsh water in Hawaii. There are many varieties found in the grocery store, but the one that is most efficacious also happens to be the cheapest. This is the golden or yellow bulb onion that is generally two and one-half to three inches in diameter and shaped something like a turnip.

Dry onions are not often successfully grown by the home gardener in Hawaii. The plant tends to grow tops in cool weather and form bulbs in warm weather, but just as important is the length of daylight. Nearly ideal conditions exist on the island of Maui in the Kula district where onions are grown commercially.

The entire bulb is used in medicine.

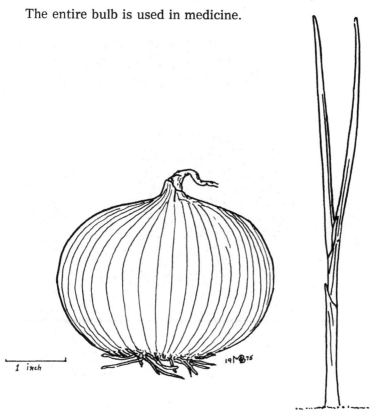

1 inch

'ALAEA

Red ferruginous ocher

'*Alaea* is a red earth composed of iron oxides found chiefly on Wai-'ale'ale on the island of Kauai. It is also found on Molokai and Maui in isolated areas and some road cuts. On the Big Island of Hawaii it is found in association with sulfur deposits and has been reported from one location in the Kohala district.

The principal use for '*alaea* today is for coloring Hawaiian salt, although in the past it was used in making a kind of red paint, for dye and also in medicine. The use of this natural iron oxide in medicinal practice is often ascribed to the so called "law of signatures," in which the color or shape of the plant or other material suggests a use, e.g. red earth to build red blood. Coincidentally, perhaps, modern medicine prescribes iron compounds for similar ailments.

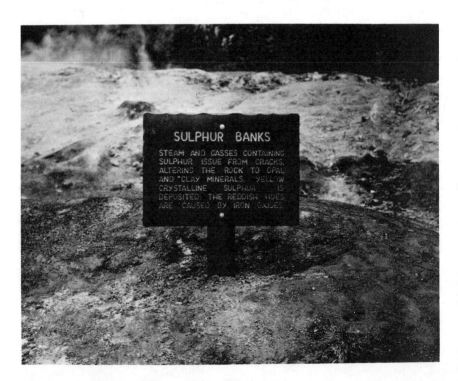

SULPHUR BANKS

STEAM AND GASSES CONTAINING SULPHUR ISSUE FROM CRACKS, ALTERING THE ROCK TO OPAL AND 'CLAY MINERALS. YELLOW CRYSTALLINE SULPHUR IS DEPOSITED. THE REDDISH HUES ARE CAUSED BY IRON OXIDES.

Red earth is sometimes found near sulfur deposits.   Photo by National Park Service.

ALOE
Aloe barbadensis syn. vera

The true *aloe* is a rosette-shaped plant with a very short stem composed of fleshy leaves that are opposite when young but mature to a complete spiral. The thick pale green leaves may grow to a foot or two long and taper from two to three inches wide at the base to a pointed tip. The leaves are narrow but stiff with spiny edges. In the center of the plant a thin stem about three feet tall bears yellowish flowers an inch long. Another Hawaiian name for aloe is *panini 'awa'awa*.

Both the agave and sisal resemble the aloe, but as mature plants are much larger. The leaves of the sisal are generally smooth-edged, ending in a purple spine. Agave or century plant has leaves three to six feet long that are widest in the middle and a flower stalk that rises 20 to 30 feet high.

Though *aloe* is native to the North African desert, it will grow well as a house plant. It seems to thrive on very little sunlight and not much water.

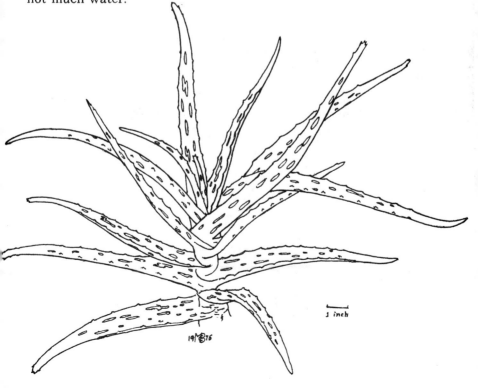

1 inch

'AMA'UMA'U

Sadleria cyatheoides

The 'ama'uma'u is one of the larger ferns found in the mountains. At optimum conditions it will have a trunk over five feet tall and seven inches in diameter, with fronds lifting eight to ten feet above the ground. The fronds are dark green and leathery on the upper side and lighter underneath. These range in size from two to three feet long by 12 to 18 inches wide. To the newcomer the 'ama-'uma'u might be confused with the true tree fern hapu'u *(cibotium splendens)* or its "brother" *hapu'u 'i'i (cibotium chamissoi)*. Since a full grown 'ama'uma'u is often larger than a young *hapu'u* of either species, the easiest way to tell them apart instantly is by the fronds themselves. The 'ama'uma'u has only a midrib with the leaflets on either side. The *hapu'u* on the other hand looks as though it had been composed of 'ama'uma'u fronds symetrically arranged along a larger stem.

'Ama'uma'u is common on the heights of all the islands, ranging from very wet to very dry conditions. Frequently the young fronds are red.

The trunk must be split to get at the pith which is then removed and sun-dried under arid conditions.

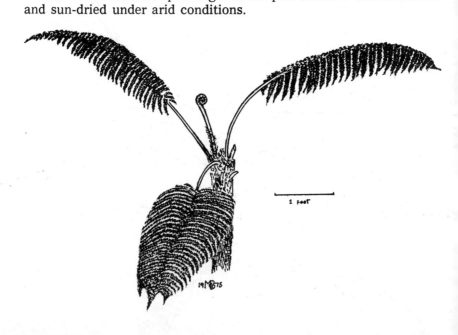

1 foot

'APE

Alocasia macrorrhiza

'Ape looks like a gigantic *taro* or *kalo* plant with huge heart-shaped leaves that may grow to be four feet long and over two feet wide. In contrast to those of *taro*, the leaves of 'ape tend to point upward adding to its height. The leaves are supported by substantial stems that rise more than four feet above a ringed trunk. The stems of 'ape may be green or a whitish color.

In the lowlands 'ape is found growing wild on the steep slopes of ravines and near old habitation sites in dry sections of the islands.

The juice from the fresh cut stems is the part of the plant that is used for medicine. Never chew a piece of any part of the uncooked 'ape plant. Tiny crystals within the organic structure can cause severe pain to the tongue and gums and may constrict the throat dangerously.

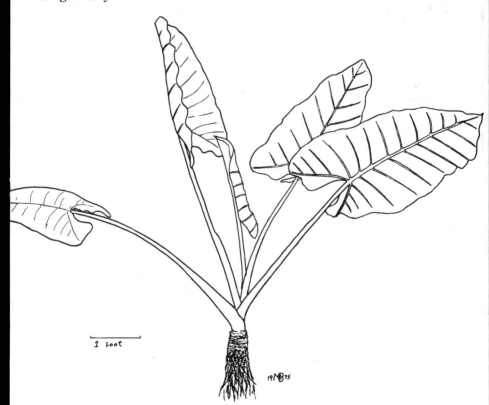

1 foot

AUHUHU

Tephrosia purpurea

Auhuhu is a short shrub seldom more than a foot and a half tall. It is a legume with a rather woody stem and thin branches containing four to seven pairs of leaflets. The small leaflets up to an inch long are smooth on top and hairy underneath. Spikes up to a foot in length support little white or purplish flowers and narrow pods up to an inch and a half long which contain four to eight seeds. When the pods mature the two sides twist open in a distinctive manner.

This herb is found growing wild in dry soil near the seashore. The leaves, which are the part of the plant used for medicine, should be gathered fresh each time they are needed. At lower altitudes *auhuhu* can be grown in the garden or in pots under conditions approximating its natural circumstances.

This plant is often called *auhola* or *hola* when it is to be used for catching fish. The leaves contain tephrosin which is said to be poisonous to fish but not to mammals.

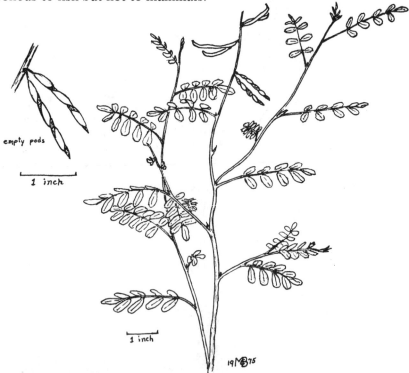

empty pods

1 inch

1 inch

19 M3 75

'AWA

Piper methysticum

'Awa is a shrub that grows up to 12 feet in height with green stems that are interrupted with swollen joints. The rather smooth, shiny leaves are a rounded heart shape seldom as large as a man's hand. About a dozen prominent veins spread out from the base of the leaf, which is attached by a short petiole.

In former times more than a dozen varieties of 'awa were recognized and named. Each was distinguished by the length of the internode, the color and the potency of the brew made from it. Once cultivated widely on all islands by the Hawaiians, it is now used as an ornamental in some gardens and found growing wild in lowland forests.

A rainy day is said to be the best for obtaining the 'awa root, which is the part of the plant used for medicine. When the ground is wet the root can be removed more easily and, if the stalk is cut into foot lengths and stuck right side up in the moist earth, new plants will grow.

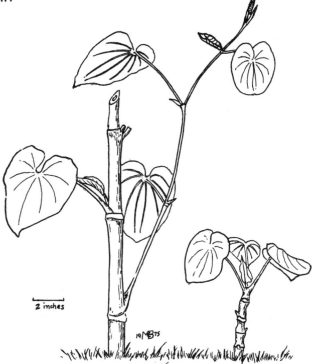

2 inches

'AWAPUHI

Zingiber zerumbet

'Awapuhi is a native wild ginger with thin narrow leaves that grow around a fleshy stem one to two feet high. The 10 or 12 leaves are arranged alternately along opposite sides of the stem and seldom exceed six or seven inches in length.

'Awapuhi grows in extensive patches in the damp open forest at lower altitudes. The root of the herb is a rhizome which branches and grows horizontally under the soil and sends up not only the leaf stalk but a separate flower stem as well. The foot-high flower stem developes late in the summer, supporting a club-like head two to three inches long, consisting of reddish to green overlapping scales covered with a slimy fluid. Only one or two flowers appear at a time.

The root is the part of the plant used for medicine. If it is stored in an open place that is rather dark and cool it will keep for some time and be available for use when needed.

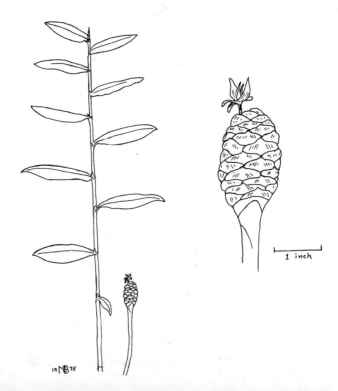

1 inch

'AWAPUHI KE'OKE'O

Hedychium coronarium

'Awapuhi ke'oke'o is the common white ginger found growing in damp open forest at altitudes up to 4,000 feet. This plant is larger than the native *'awapuhi*, standing three to four feet high with leaves up to 20 inches long and up to four inches wide. The conspicuous characteristic is the white fragrant flower which is produced in groups on the same stem as the leaves.

This herb can be cultivated easily with only a little care and used not only as an attractive ornamental but the flowers can be used as medicine. A cool, wet location with adequate soil and partial shade seems to produce the most vigorous plants.

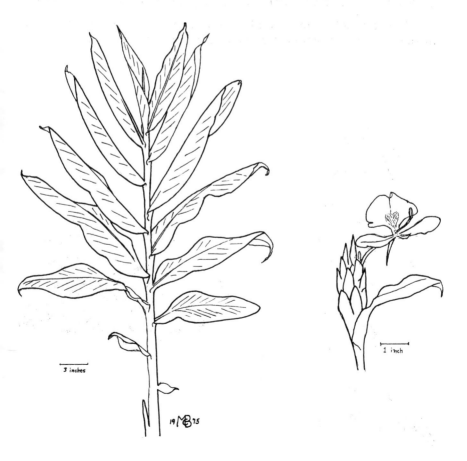

3 inches

1 inch

19 MB 75

'AWAPUHI PAKE

Zingiber officinale

'Awapuhi pake, often called Chinese ginger root, can be cultivated up to an altitude of 2,000 feet or more under the right conditions. It is similar to the 'awapuhi but reaches two to four feet. It also differs in having narrower, smooth leaves and yellowish green and purple flowers.

In Hawaii the root is sun-dried for commercial purpose and used either dried or green for flavoring food and the green root for making candied ginger.

The 'awapuhi pake root planted from a budded root takes about a year to mature. When the leaves wither it is ready to harvest.

'Awapuhi pake can generally be purchased in any grocery store in the islands. The roots keep well in a cool dry place.

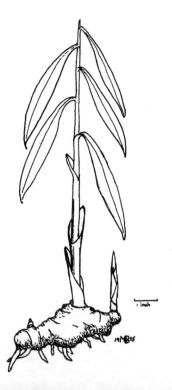

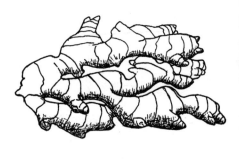

HAPU'U
Cibotium splendens

The *hapu'u* is the most common tree fern in Hawaii. In the rain forest the trunk often reaches 16 feet in height under optimum conditions, with the fronds lifting eight to ten feet above that. This fern is widely cultivated as an ornamental and as a shade for some flowers, but does not grow so large as in the wild state.

The frond of *hapu'u* consists of a main stem with pairs of branchlets arranged on either side. The under portion of the leaflets are light green to whitish, often giving a frosty appearance at night.

Hapu'u is sometimes confused with a similar species called *hapu'u i'i* (cibotium chamissoi). They are most easily told apart by the appearance of the stems. *Hapu'u i'i* stems are adorned with blackish bristles. By contrast the stems of *hapu'u* are smooth, although when young they may be covered with a brownish, silky material called *pulu*. It is this *pulu* and scrapings from the green stem below it that are used for medicine.

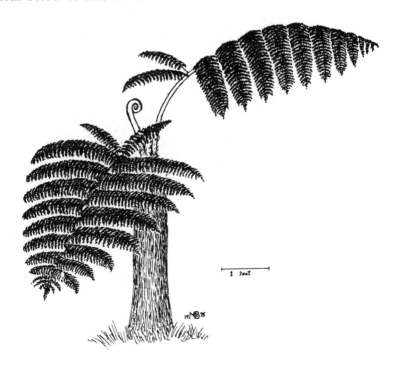

1 foot

HAU

Hibiscus tiliaceus

The *hau* tree grows near the seacoast where it sometimes forms a jungle of reclining trunks and interwoven branches that take root wherever they touch ground. Occasionally it may become a tree of medium height with a crooked trunk and twisted branches. The rounded, heart-shaped leaves vary from two inches to a foot in diameter. They are somewhat leathery with a smooth surface, while the underside is velvety white.

The distinguishing feature and the part of the tree used for medicine is the large yellow flower on or near the ends of the branches. It is two to three inches long and when opening has a sulfur yellow color, sometimes having a dark red center. As the day proceeds, the yellow gives way to orange and by dark, changes to reddish brown.

The *hau* tree may be cultivated up to about 2000 feet.

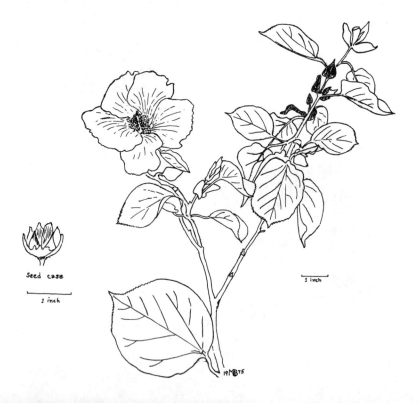

Seed case

1 inch

1 inch

HA'UOI

Verbina litoralis

Ha'uoi or owi is a moderately fast growing weed two to three feet tall that may reach a height of six feet under optimum conditions. It has thin, smooth stems that are four-sided. The leaves are narrow and pointed, one and one-half to two and one-half inches long with course-toothed margins. This freely branching herb produces tiny blue flowers at the ends of long slender stalks.

Ha'uoi seems to grow best in the leeward sections between 2000 and 7000 feet in altitude, but can be found on all the islands in any open area that is not too dry.

All of the green parts of this plant are used for making medicine. If there are no plants growing naturally nearby, it would be desirable to relocate some specimens to a convenient area.

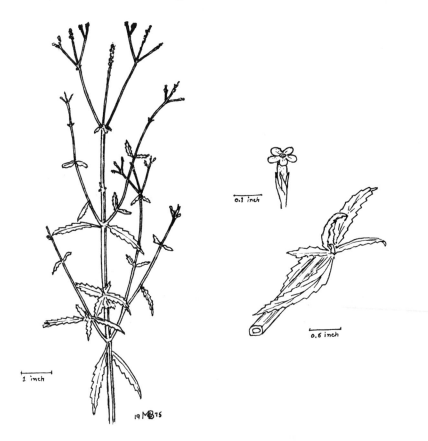

0.1 inch

0.6 inch

1 inch

HINU HONU

Turtle oil

Hinu Honu (turtle oil) is obtained from the same green turtle *chelonia mydas* that is often used for food. This animal attains a maximum length of close to four feet. It is distinguished from other sea turtles by the horny plates of the back which do not overlap but meet edge to edge.

These turtles are most easily captured at night on secluded sandy beaches when they are returning to the sea after laying their eggs. Before hunting the turtle one must obtain a free permit from the Division of Fish and Game of the State of Hawaii, and become acquainted with the following restrictions:.

Turtles may be taken only for home consumption, by using a spear or by hand. Using a net is forbidden. Each captured animal must measure 36 inches across the shell.

Turtle oil is procured by cooking the fat and expressing the oil from it. The finished product will keep almost indefinitely if refrigerated.

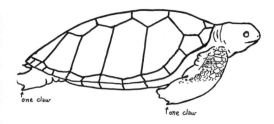

one claw

one claw

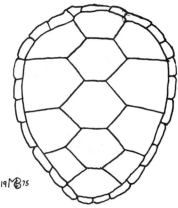

NOTICE

Since September 6, 1978, a ban on the taking of sea turtles of any size has been in effect.

The author recommends trying any organic oil for some treatments until the green sea turtle is removed from the endangered list.

HOʻIʻO

Athyrium arnottii

Hoʻiʻo is a large fern restricted to the mountainous areas of Hawaii. The fronds are large and complex, often three or four feet long, and coarser than those of the *akolea*. Spore dots are abundant on the underside of the mature fronds. Below the branches the midribs are dark brown and smooth, but are covered with dark scales at the bases.

The *hoʻiʻo* fern is commonly found in the moist shady areas of the mountains. It will not grow at low altitudes. The young fronds are gathered as an article of food to be eaten raw with salted salmon or freshwater shrimp. Sometimes bundles of the young shoots can be found for sale in some markets.

The young fronds are gathered and dried to be used for medicine.

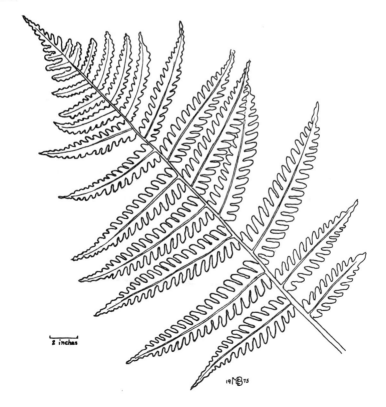

2 inches

19MB75

IHI

Oxalis corniculata

Ihi is a creeping perennial herb commonly found growing among lawn grasses in acid soil. The three leaflets rise on a slender stem two or three inches high. They are an inverted heart shape, forming a triad that would fit within a one inch circle. This plant can easily be distinguished from clover by the pleasant sour taste of the leaves and by the way the leaflets fold down against the stem at night.

The tiny, yellow, well-shaped flowers occur at the top of slender stalks. A related species called *ihi makole* has orange flowers and red stems. The leaves of both plants are used in medicine.

Ingestion of large amounts of *ihi* might be poisonous due to the presence of oxalic acid.

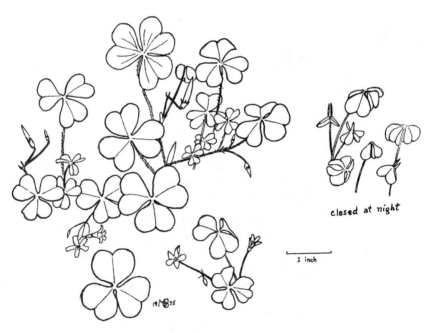

closed at night

1 inch

ILIOHE
Moss

Iliohe is a dark green moss that grows in fresh water and is often found in the cool waters of springs and streams. The colonies of this plant present a rounded appearance, much the same as the rocks among which they grow. In the water *iliohe* feels soft and velvety but when it begins to dry it is harsh to the touch.

This moss is used both in the green state and dried for medicine. It should be washed very well to remove all foreign material and then may be dried directly in the sun. When *iliohe* is partly dry it can be broken **apart** easily which will hasten the process of drying.

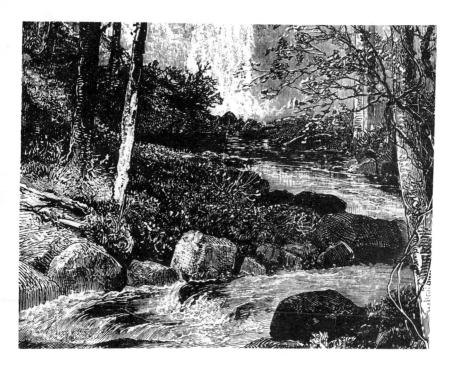

ILIE'E

Plumbago zeylanica

Ilie'e is a relatively short shrub seldom growing more than three feet high. A single rootstock supports numerous slender, green fluted stems with branches spreading sideways up to a foot in length. The thin, rather rough leaves are virtually stemless ovals or oblongs up to three inches long. The leaves are whitish on the underside and have smooth to wavy margins. Right after a rain the same branches produce white tubular flowers less than an inch long at the branch ends.

Ilie'e is found in the dry areas near the seashore on all of the islands. The plant seems to thrive in harsh conditions of hard soil among rocks. The root is dug and preserved in a relatively fresh condition for use in medicine.

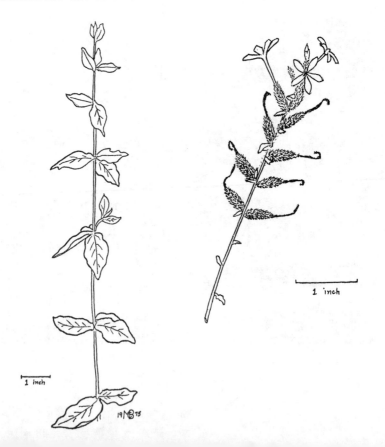

1 inch

1 inch

INIKO

Indigofera suffruticosa

Iniko is a legume with many branches which grows to height of three to five feet. The compound leaves are composed of a terminal leaflet and two to eight pairs on a petiole three to six inches long. The thin leaflets are pointed oblongs ranging from one-half to one and one-half inches in length that are paler green on the underside. Many small reddish flowers develop on spikes at the base of the petiole. These in time become clusters of tiny curved pods about one-half inch long, each of which contains three to eight minute reddish-black seeds.

Iniko is found on all of the islands, inhabiting the rather dry pasture lands and open forest below 3,000 feet in elevation.

Care should be exercised in gathering the leaves which are used for medicine since they have miniscule sharp hairs on them which can cause an itch or a rash on those who are sensitive.

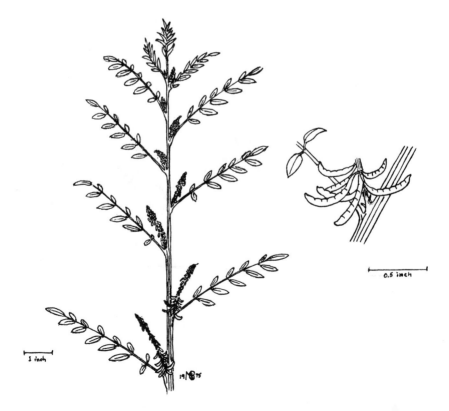

0.5 inch

1 inch

IPU 'AWA'AWA

Lagenaria siceraria

The *ipu 'awa'awa* is a variety of bottle gourd with bitter tasting pulp. The plant is a vine with downy branched tendrils, bearing leaves that are a rounded heart shape. The leaves which range in size from four inches to over a foot wide are downy to hairy. A distinctive feature of this plant is that the single white flowers bloom at night. The hard-shelled fruit varies considerably in size and shape with each variety.

The fruit of *ipu 'awa'awa* is extremely bitter. Perhaps the easiest way to insure getting the correct variety is to ask a knowledgeable Hawaiian to help you locate a plant or possibly to give you some seed.

Both the young and the mature fruit are used as medicine, as are the young tendrils and leaves.

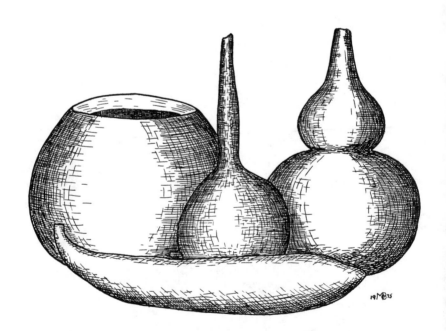

KO

Saccharum officinarum

Ko is the most common commercial plant in Hawaii. Sugar cane grows best at low elevations but has been cultivated at an altitude near 3,000 feet.

The sugar cane grown today is a hybrid of many varieties. The jointed stalks, an inch thick, grow 15 to 20 feet tall. The foot long leaves are narrow and have a saw tooth edge. After about two years the stem produces a featherlike silver tassel which signals the plants maturity.

The old Hawaiians recognized at least 40 varieties of *ko*, but only a few were used for medicine. *Kokea* was a native cane with a greenish-yellow stem and a thin rind that was easily removed or crushed. Perhaps because of this, the sweet juice of *kokea* was popular as an ingredient in medicine.

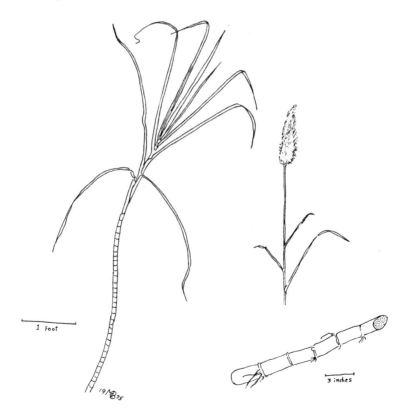

1 Foot

3 inches

KOA

Acacia koa

No tree in Hawaii gains a greater size than the *koa*. The largest trees may be 60 to 80 feet to the first limbs and more than 10 feet in diameter. The *koa* grows best in the damp forest between 1,500 and 5,000 feet altitude. At places where this tree has matured alone the branches are low, twisted and bearded with gray lichen.

Other than size, the most distinctive feature of this legume is its having two different kinds of leaves. When the plant is just a few feet tall it has tiny leaflets one-fourth to one-half inch long, arranged in pairs along pinnae which in turn are paired on a petiole or steam. As the tree ages, the petiole flattens out and becomes curved, while the primitive leaves drop off. The remaining sickle-shaped "leaf" and the bark are the parts of the *koa* used for medicine.

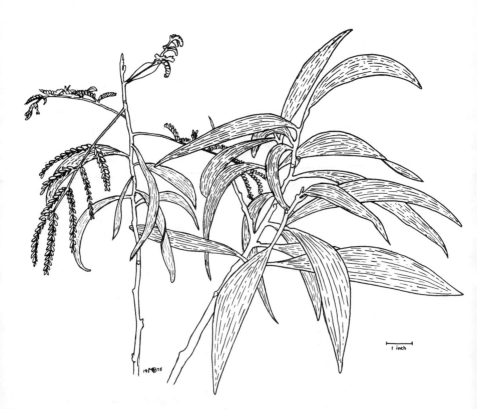

1 inch

KOALI

Ipomoea Sp.

There are two kinds of *koali* or morning glory that are used for medicine. *Koali 'awa (ipomoea congesta)* is very common from the seashore to over 2,000 feet in altitude, wherever it can grow unshaded. This vine bears heart-shaped leaves several inches long and bell-shaped flowers that open in the morning and close in the evening. When they open the flowers are blue, but slowly change to pink as the day progresses.

Pohuehue (ipomoea pes-caprae) is a morning glory that grows just above the high water line on sandy beaches. It is a smooth green vine that roots at the joints with broad rounded leaves, notched at the end. The bell-shaped flower is pink and may be single or in clusters.

The entire *koali* plant is gathered fresh for medicine.

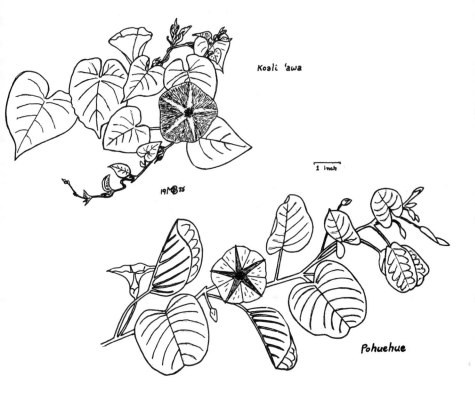

Koali 'awa

1 inch

Pohuehue

KO'OKO'OLAU

Bidens Spp.

Ko'oko'olau is a many branched native shrub seldom growing more than three feet high. A woody stem supports slender green branches each with three to five pairs of leaves. The pointed oval leaves are two to four inches long and one to two inches wide with a stem nearly half as long as the leaf. The leaves are thin and smooth with a toothed margin. As new leaves are produced at the branch ends, the older pairs below turn yellow and droop. Most fall but some may dry and hang on the plant if undisturbed. The yellowish flowers give way to narrow barbed seeds nearly one-half inch long that are called Spanish needles.

Similar plants introduced from tropical America *(Bidens pilosa)* also have burs called Spanish needles. They also grow at lower elevations on all islands. The fresh young shoots of this imported weed are gathered for a tea named *kinehe* but it is the brew made from the leaves of *ko'oko'olau* that is used for medicine. A cup of *ko'oko'olau* tea in the morning is particularly good for reviving a failing appetite, and regular use is said to prevent a stroke.

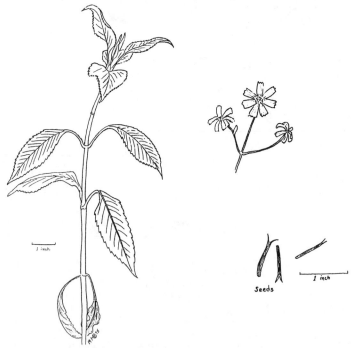

1 inch

Seeds

1 inch

KUAWA

Psidium guajava

Kuawa is a shrub or tree introduced into Hawaii from tropical America before 1800. It grows so well at lower elevations that in some places it has formed dense thickets. The tree seldom exceeds a height of 20 feet and in dry areas it may remain a spreading shrub less than four feet tall. The reddish-brown bark sometimes sloughs off, exposing the green inner bark, which gives the trunk and branches a mottled appearance.

The leaves are oval-shaped, rather rough and three to six inches long. The inch-wide flowers are white and somewhat fragrant. The most distinguishing feature is the fruit which is about the size and shape of a lemon. The rind is thick, protecting a deep pink pulp which contains dark caviar-like seeds.

The leaf buds are the part of the *kuawa* used for medicine.

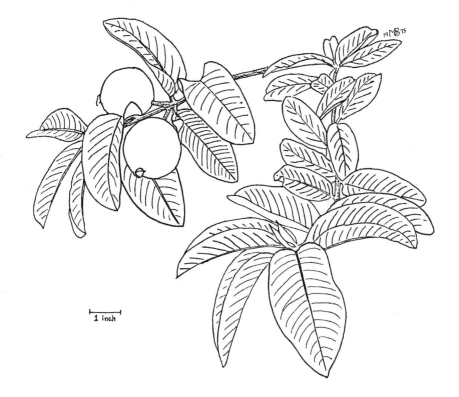

1 inch

KUKUI

Aleurites moluccana

The *kukui* tree is characterized by light green foliage which makes it easy to pick out from a distance. Generally, *kukui* grows about 50 feet tall, but some trees are known which are almost twice as high. The leaves resemble those of the maple, having generally three lobes but on some leaves the lobes are only suggested and they appear as a long pointed oval. Larger leaves may be seven to nine inches long and five to seven inches wide with a grayish underside. The small white flowers are clustered at the branch ends. The fruit is a green irregular ball two inches in diameter on a stem three or four inches long.

Kukui is a common tree at elevations below 2000 feet and is frequently found near ancient house sites. It grows well on cliff sides and in gulches at the lowest elevations.

The bark, flowers and nuts are all used for medicine.

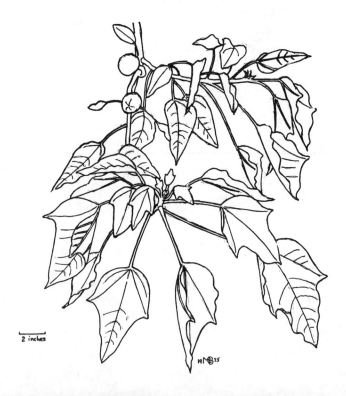

2 inches

LAPINE

Cymbopogon citratus

Lapine is an oil grass which originated in southern Asia. Whenever this grass is cut or crushed, the leaves release a pleasant scent which is reminiscent of the zest of lemons.

This grass grows in tufts, producing pointed green blades two to three feet long and three-fourths to one inch wide. In common with many cutting grasses, *lapine* possesses a microscopic sawtooth margin that can cause "paper" cuts on the skin of the careless.

Lapine has been in the islands for a long time. Some families have literally handed down plants from generation to generation. The best way to obtain a start is to ask a Hawaiian friend or one from the Philippines for it. *Lapine* is often cultivated in well-drained patches or in pots to serve as an ornamental and at the same time to have it available to use in medicine.

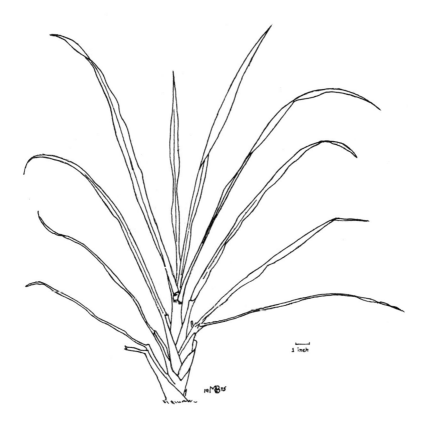

1 inch

LIMU KAHA
Liverwort Spp.

Limu kaha is a mossly kind of primitive plant which resembles a mat of short pieces of very dark green ribbon. It grows flat over rocks and is often found spreading out on the walls at the entrances of wet to damp lava tubes. *Limu kaha* also inhabits the shady sides of cliffs which are particularly wet.

This plant is used in the fresh state for medicine. It is harvested by sliding a flat blade-like spatula between it and the rock. It sould be washed in fresh water to remove all foreign materials.

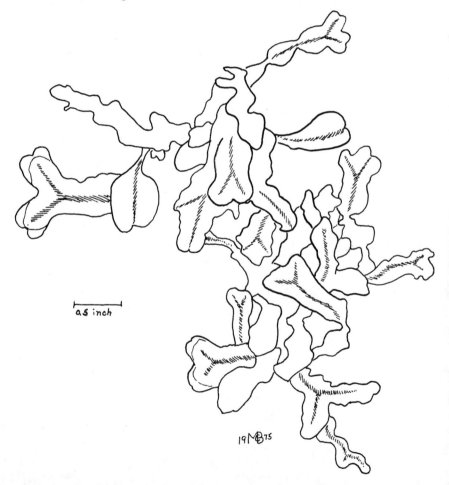

0.5 inch

19 MB 75

LAU-KAHI
Plantago major

Lau-kahi is a broadleafed plant common to lawns and pasture lands. Because this herb grows without a stem it frequently is missed by the lawn mower and by grazing animals. The leaves are a broad oval in shape and form on a rosette that is low to or horizontal with the ground. The leaf blades range in size from one to nine inches in length, with several prominent veins extending from the tip to the trough-shaped leaf stem.

Flowers are borne on a slender spike that rises four to twelve inches above the leaves. When the seeds mature the stalk resembles a head of grain.

Lau-kahi is found from lowlands not far from the sea to an altitude exceeding 3,000 feet. Some varieties may range even higher. The leaves of all are gathered for medicine.

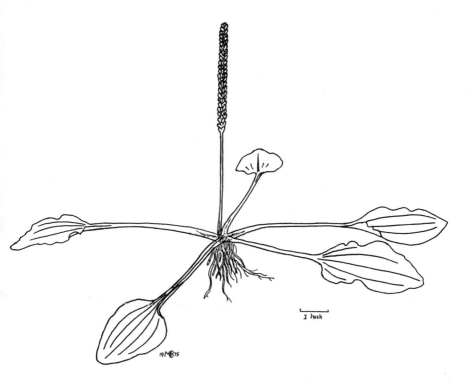

1 Inch

MIKANA
Carica papaya

The *mikana* or papaya tree has a very primitive appearance. The young trees especially are unbranched, with stems and leaves crowningf the gently tapered trunk. As new stems are produced at the top, the lowest on the trunk fall off, leaving regular heart-shaped scars. The leaves are large, sometimes more than two feet wide, and are deeply lobed.

The fruit are borne on the trunk of the tree at the base of the stem and are clustered entirely around the tree, with the more mature fruits at the bottom. The fruit are oval or rounded, six inches or more long, with yellowish to orange pulp similar in texture to a melon. The mature fruit is generally yellow with a central cavity containing small black seeds.

Both the leaves and the milky sap from the skin of the green fruit are used for medicinal purpose.

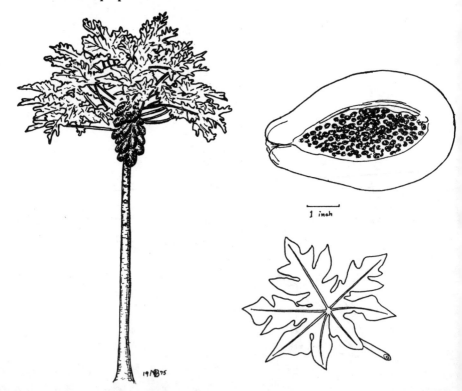

1 inch

NAUPAKA KAHAKAI
Scaevola sericea

Naupaka kahakai is a beach plant having numerous branches spreading out widely from a low base. This succulent shrub may grow to a height of eight to ten feet where it is planted for a hedge or fence. In the wild state it is more often a low angular plant less than three feet tall. The thick, fleshy leaves are clustered at the tips of the branches and are distinctive in both color and shape. The bright green leaves are three to five inches long and pear-shaped with an indented end. These and the root are the part of the plant used for medicine.

The most conspicuous feature of this shrub is the flower, which is small, white and gives the appearance of having been torn in half. The berries are white, about half of an inch long and resemble hailstones.

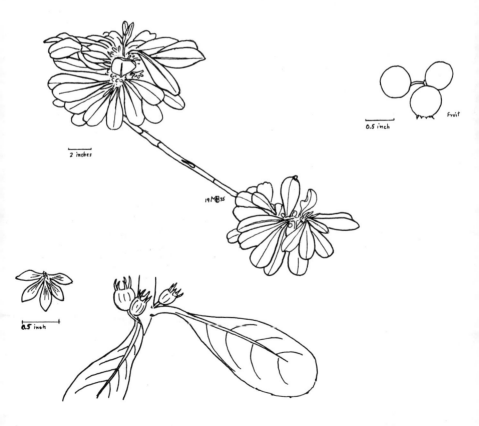

Fruit
0.5 inch

2 inches

0.5 inch

NIU

Cocos nucifera

Niu is probably the best known and most easily recognized palm tree in the world. The tree is slender with a slightly curved trunk that is thick at the base with some roots which may be above ground. The comparatively thin, ringed stem supports a multitude of fronds 10 to 18 feet long up to 90 feet above the ground.

This palm begins bearing coconuts when six to eight years old and continues to grow and fruit until it is about 70 years old, although some trees may live a full century.

The mature fruit is about the size of a football with a tendency to having three sides. A thick fibrous husk encases the hard-shelled nut which has three pores on the end. One pore may be easily punched in to obtain the coconut water which, along with the white meat inside, is used for medicine.

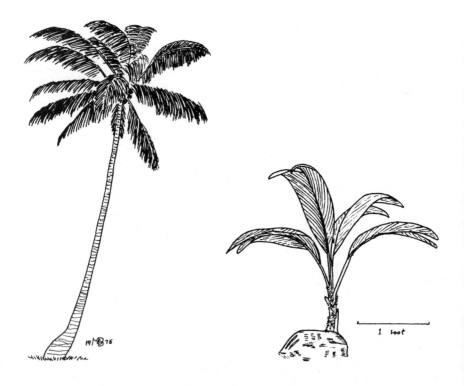

1 foot

NONI

Morinda citrafolia

Noni is a small tree or shrub with shiny, dark green leaves on greenish, angular branches. As a tree *noni* seldom exceeds 10 feet in height but may grow half again that high in ideal circumstances. The oval leaves are thick and deep veined, seven to nine inches long and three to four inches wide. The leaves are generally paired, although one leaf is sometimes replaced by flower heads which grow to become mature fruit three to four inches long and two to four inches in diameter. The fruits resemble those of the breadfruit, only smaller, having the surface divided into polygonal cells. The *noni* fruit is pale yellow and has an unpleasant taste and a foul odor.

In former times *noni* figured in many medicines. It is often found growing near ancient house sites between the shore and the lowland woods. The juice of very ripe *noni* was used in the treatment of diabetes, heart trouble and high blood pressure. The juice was diluted with water and used as a drink before meals and resting periods.

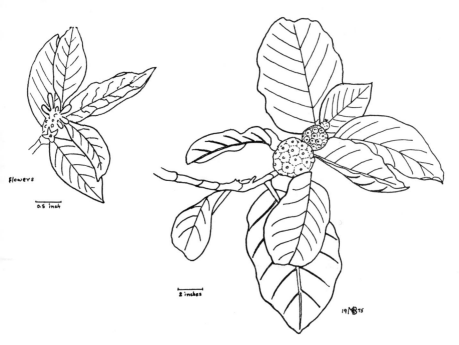

flowers

0.5 inch

2 inches

OHELO KAU LA'AU

Vaccinium calycinum

Ohelo kau la'au is a brittle, woody shrub that may grow to a height of 10 feet where supported by surrounding trees. The leaves are relatively thin pointed ovals two to four inches long with prominent veins and a fine toothed margin. The most conspicuous characteristic is the small red fruits which are consistent in color in contrast to those of the common *ohelo* (*V. retculatum*). These berries are easily distinguished from those of *akia* by having many tiny seeds.

The *ohelo kau la'au* can be found in the open rain forest of the uplands on the larger islands of the Hawaiian group.

The tart berries are the part of the plant gathered for medicinal use. The juice can be expressed and frozen into ice cubes for subsequent use when needed. The juice of this *ohelo* is said to be particularly good for the treatment of bladder and kidney disorders.

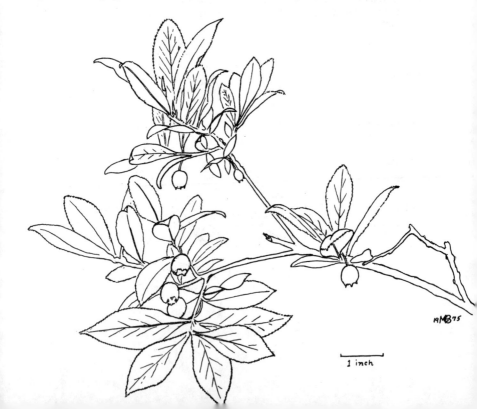

1 inch

OHIA LEHUA
Metrosideros collina Subsp. polymorpha

Ohia lehua ranges in size from a shrub several inches high, found in swamps on Kauai, to huge trees a hundred feet high in the forests of Hawaii. The appearance of this plant is just as variable as its size. The leaves may be pointed, oval, round or narrow and can be smooth or downy on the underside. Young leaves may be light green, pink or red and mature ones gray-green to dark green. The tree may be thick and spreading in the open and tall and thin where competition is keen. The bark varies from furrowed to shaggy to smooth.

The many varieties or forms of *ohia lehua* all share one thing in common. The flowers are conspicuous, feathery blooms made up of many tufts up to one and one-half inches long. However, even the flowers or different plants vary in color, size and shape. They range from scarlet, pink, orange, yellow to white and may be single, double or multiple blooms of densely packed stamens.

The bark of *ohia lehua* trees and the young shoots with red leaves are gathered for medicine.

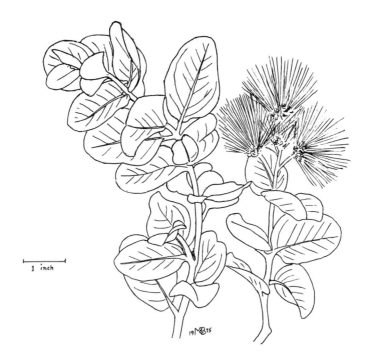

1 inch

OLAPA

Cheirodendron guadichaudii

Olapa is one of the commonest trees in the upland forest. Its bright green leaves are in constant motion in the slightest breeze, which distinguishes it even at a distance. This evergreen grows to a height of 20 to 30 feet with relatively few angular branches. The bark is smooth and mottled or banded with colors ranging from light gray and greenish gray to nearly black. The rather coarse branches are marked with leaf scars and are green or yellowish green near the leaf ends. The leaves are generally opposite with long stems which are tough and flexible, permitting the leaflets to flutter ceaselessly. The leaves are palmately divided into two to five leaflets which are smooth and leathery with occasional serrations along the margin. The leaflets are from two to seven inches long and one and one-half to five inches wide and pointed oblongs to ovals and are trough-shape rather than flat. The cluster of greenish flowers on the branch ends are in time replaced by drupes of small black berries. The root of *olapa* is dug up for medicine.

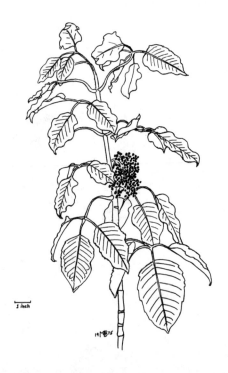

1 inch

OLIWA-KU-KAHAKAI
Bryophyllum pinnatum

Oliwa-ku-kahakai is an air plant that generally grows to a height of two to three feet, but may reach six feet in ideal circumstances. The variegated, reddish stem supports thick, fleshy leaves and purplish-green cylindrical flowers which hang like oriental lanterns. The oval, scalloped leaves are two to four inches long and one to two inches wide. They are generally paired on opposite sides of the stem but may be three to five parted.

A distinguishing characteristic of this succulent herb is its method of propagation. When a leaf is detached and placed in a damp location, a score of tiny plants begin to grow from the notches in the leaf margins.

The plant thrives in rather dry waste places on all of the islands. It grows well in thin rocky soil below 2,000 feet elevation but may be cultivated at higher altitudes. The leaves of this herb are gathered fresh for medicine.

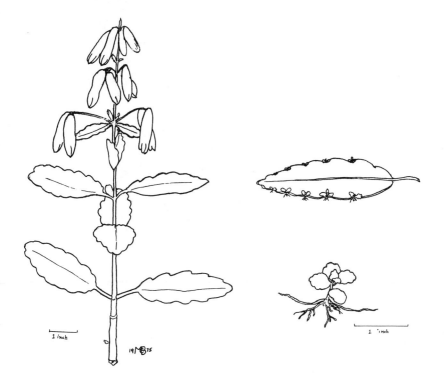

1 inch

1 inch

PAKIKAWAIO

Cyclosorus (Dryopteris) cyatheoides

Pakikawaio is a large fern found in the uplands forest. It stands three or more feet high on relatively slender, long dark stems. The fronds may be two to four feet long and six to sixteen inches wide. The frond is oblong in shape, with a terminal pinna that is quite similar to the pairs opposing each other on the stem. Each frond may consist of 10 to 24 pairs of narrow, toothed pinnae. These oblong pinnae are from one-half to one-fifth of the length.

The fresh root is the part of the plant that is gathered for medicine.

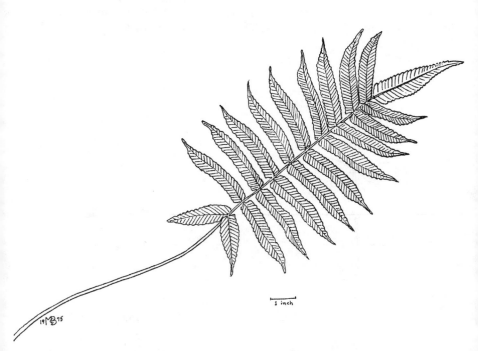

1 inch

PALEPIWA

Eucalyptus Spp.

Palepiwa (ward off fever) is the Hawaiian name for all eucalyptus trees. About 50 species have been introduced into the islands from Australia, but only about a fifth of these can be considered common. These trees grow very rapidly and some species attain a height of over 300 feet, thus ranking as the tallest plants in Hawaii.

Young shoots of *palepiwa* may have bluish leaves that are opposite, heart-shaped and stemless. These give way to the typical alternate leathery leaves with a smooth margin as the trees age. The thick leaves tend to hang vertically or obliquely and some species have a marked citrus or peppermint odor. The red or whitish feathery flowers hang in clusters and produce a woody cup-shaped receptacle containing many tiny seeds. The bark of various species differs considerably. Some are thick and grooved, others rough, while a few are very smooth with patches flaking off, presenting a mottled green, gray and brown appearance. Leaves of all varieties are used in medicine.

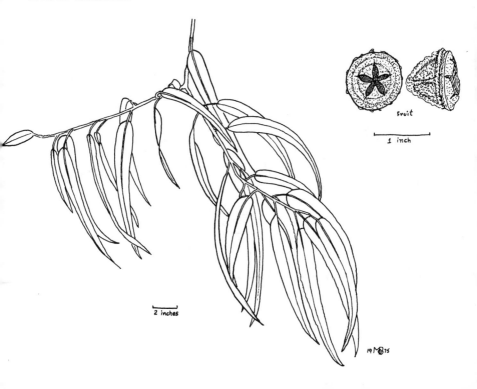

fruit

1 inch

2 inches

PEPA OR PAPERBARK

Melaleluca laucadendra

The most conspicuous feature of this tree is the numerous layers of bark which peel away from the trunk. This paper bark is gray to light tan in color and the spongy layers are easily removed.

The leaves of this tree are alternate, long ovals in shape and may be slightly curved. The veins are parallel the length of the leaf which is two to six inches long. The flower resembles a *lehua* or a bottle brush and ranges in color from white to pink.

Pepa was brought to Hawaii from Australia and has long been used in reforestation projects. As a consequence, some of the trees are of large size. It is easier to collect leaves from the shorter specimens. These are gathered fresh when needed to be used as medicine.

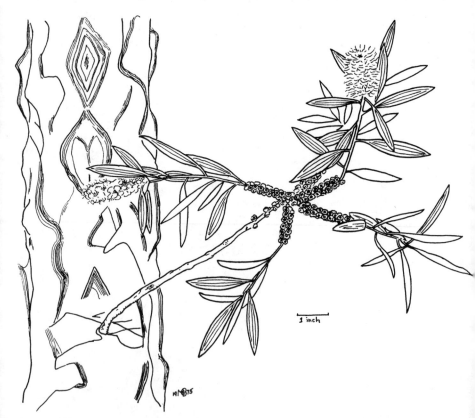

PIA

Tacca leontopetaloides

Pia is the Hawaiian name for arrowroot from which fine starch is made. It is now a rare plant but is cultivated as an ornamental in some gardens and can still be found in isolated places in the wild. This herb is an annual, sending up a leaf stalk in the spring from a tuber that is dormant during the winter. The plant grows one to three feet high with slender, fine fluted stems supporting palmately divided leaves which are reminiscent of *papaya* foliage. The many-lobed leaves are one to two feet wide with the veins depressed on the upper surface of the leaf and in bold relief on the underside. The under surface is shiny with the veins yellow.

Pia grows best in open woods near running water in a warm but somewhat shady environment. It is suggested that instead of gathering a number of tubers for medicine an entire plant be relocated for future use.

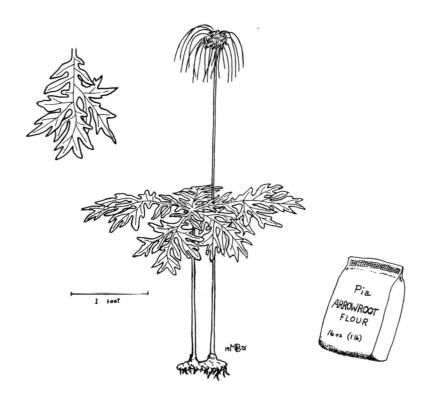

PI'IPI'I-LAU-MANAMANA

Asplenium lobulatum

Pi'ipi'i-lau-manamana (crinkled appendages) is an attractive native fern with narrow fronds up to one and one-half feet long. It has many narrow lobes like crinkled fingers along opposite sides of the axis. The stalk or axis is fairly stiff and may be reddish in color.

This fern may be found throughout a fairly wide range in altitudes where there is an abundance of moisture. The larger variety thrives in the damp jungle and around the entrances to lava tubes. A smaller variety called *anali'i* (stunted) inhabits gulches and shaded ravines which may have periodic drying.

The fronds of *pi'ipi'i-lau-manamana* are collected and thoroughly dried and then carefully burned to ashes which are used in medicine.

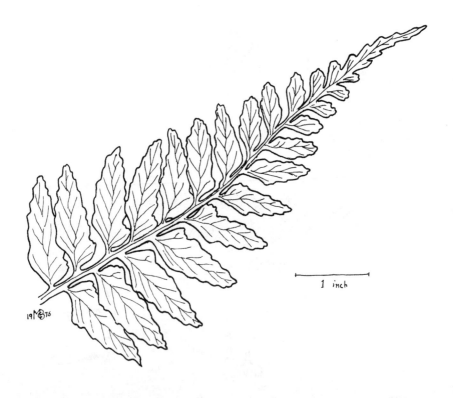

1 inch

PIPI

Psilotum complanatum

Pipi is one of two species of *psilotum* found in the islands. This primitive plant inhabits open forest from near the seacoast to over 4,000 feet elevation. It begins its growth perpendicular to the trunk of a tree or fern and then bends downward like the tail of a horse. The branches of *pipi* are flattened and notched, hanging down from the stem five inches or more.

The second species is *moa*, *(psilotum nudum)*, a slender many branched "cousin" which usually grows on the ground. It is also a leafless plant having thin, scaled green stems which function as leaves. *Moa* may grow eight to ten inches high and is characterized by branches which fork again and again.

Both *pipi* and *moa* have similar properties and may be gathered collectively to be used in medicine.

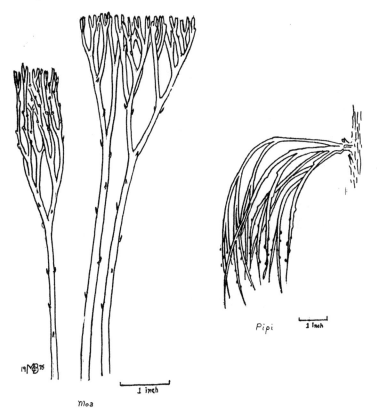

Pipi

1 Inch

moa

1 inch

POHE KULA

Centella asiatica

Pohe kula is a creeping plant with a stem one to six inches in length between joints. This herb puts down roots from each joint and sends up rosettes of long-stemmed leaves to rise above them. These petioles are up to a foot long and support leaves which are somewhat variable. Generally the leaves are rounded with a scalloped margin and one to two inches in diameter. They are deeply indented at the base something like the leaves of a violet. The flower stems range from one-half to two inches tall and are significantly shorter than those of the leaf stem, supporting tiny white flowers.

Pohe kula is commonly found at elevations below 1,500 feet, where it frequently comes up in gardens and fields as a weed. This plant has a long tap root which, along with the leaves, is used for medicine.

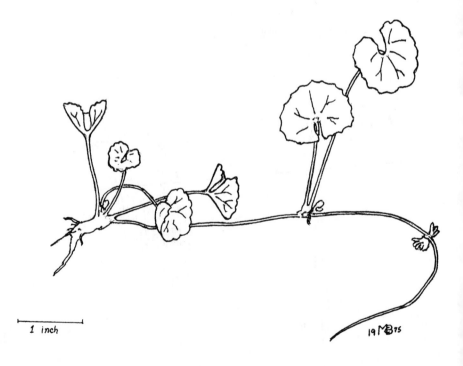

1 inch

19 MB 75

POPOLO

Solanum nigrum

Popolo is a branching green herb with a tendency to being woody at the base. This annual grows one to three feet high on cultivated land and is regarded as a common weed. The leaves may be somewhat rough and vary from youth to maturity. On the young plants the leaves are notched or slightly lobed, but as the plants mature the leaves become long oval-shaped with a wavy or indented margin.

The tiny, whitish flowers have conspicuous yellow centers and petals that may curl under. They hang in clusters and in time produce juicy, black berries about one-fourth inch in diameter.

Although the leaves of *popolo* may grow to four inches long, the smaller leaves are favored for medicine.

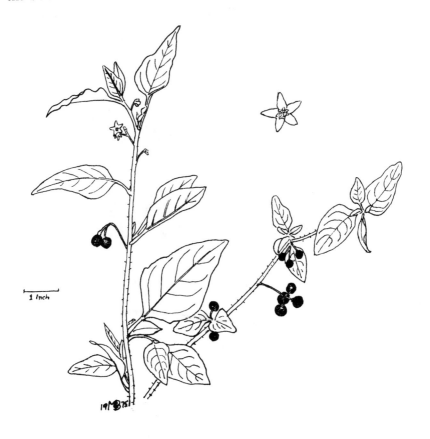

1 Inch

PUAKALA

Argemone glauca

Puakala is a prickly poppy which is native to the dryer areas of Hawaii's islands. It presents a grayish appearance except for the conspicuous white blooms which seem to occur all year around. This thistle-like plant may grow more than four feet high and is well covered with tiny sharp spines on the stem, leaves and buds. The most bothersome prickles are on the leaves which range from one to five inches long. They are irregularly lobed and toothed, embracing the stem halfway around.

The flowers produced on the branch ends are a distinctive feature of this plant, enabling it to be seen for some distance. The bloom has an orange center with a red spot in the middle of it, set in a cup of six white petals three inches in diameter.

Puakala thrives in waste places of arid rocky ground from near sea level to about 1,000 feet altitude. The entire plant is gathered fresh to use in medicine.

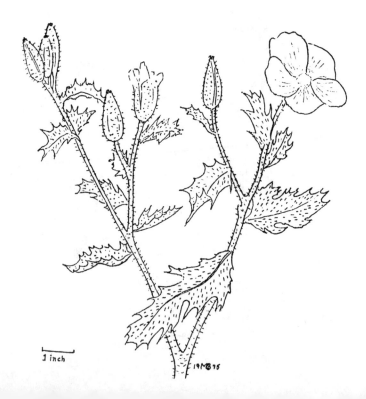

1 inch

PUA-PILIPILI

Desmodium uncinatum

Pua-pilipili is a herb that grows from one to three feet high along roads, trails and in pasture lands. Its most conspicuous feature is the chain of small flat burs that commonly adhere to clothing and the coats of some animals. Although this plant is a legume with characteristic small, whitish flowers, it has only three leaflets making up the compound leaf. The ovate leaflets are more or less smooth on top and downy to hairy underneath. They range in size from one-half to two and one-half inches long and have a noticeably lighter area along the midrib.

Pua-pilipili grows well in wet sections of all of the islands. Because of its green chains of burs that stick to clothes, this plant is regarded as a nuisance not to be encouraged near habitation. The leaves are gathered to use as medicine.

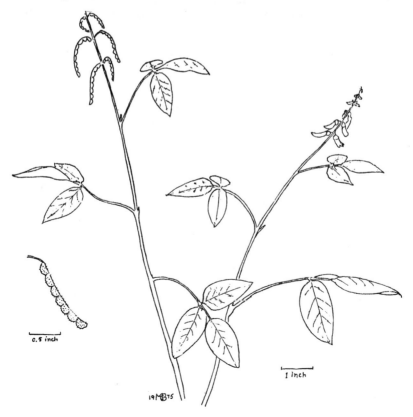

c. 5 inch

1 inch

TARO (KALO)

Colocasia esculenta

Taro is cultivated both in the uplands and in marshy land irrigated by streams. Some varieties of dry land *taro* will grow well at altitudes over 4,000 feet. The plants are perennial herbs, long grown in Hawaii for food. The long heart-shaped leaves are supported by erect stems that may be green, red, blackish or variegated. The new leaf and stem pushes out of the base of the innermost stalk, unrolling after it has emerged. Tiny plants appear around the base of the root corm.

A plant some times mistaken for *taro* is *ape (alocasia macrorrhiza.)* The latter has huge leaves that tend to point upward in contrast to *taro* blades which dip earthward.

Do not eat any part of the *taro* plant before cooking it! Chewing will express microscopic oxalic acid crystals that cause severe pain in contacted areas. All parts of the *taro* plant may be used as medicine.

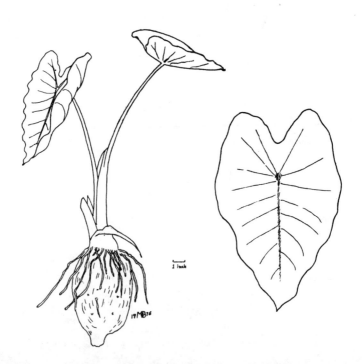

TI (KI)

Cordyline terminalis

Ti is one of the most distinctive common plants in Hawaii. Generally it has the appearance of a ringed broomstick surmounted by a feather duster of long broad green leaves. It may grow as high as 12 feet. Sometimes the *ti* plant develops branches, each of which supports a tightly spiraled leaf cluster. The leaves are smooth, shiny and very flexible, reaching a length of one to two feet and a width of five inches. As the new leaves form in the center, the old ones on the outside turn yellow and droop, eventually falling to leave a circular scar or ring.

Ti is widely cultivated from sea level to 4,000 feet altitude and may be found growing wild in wet open forest at lower elevations. The leaves of *ti* are used in medicine.

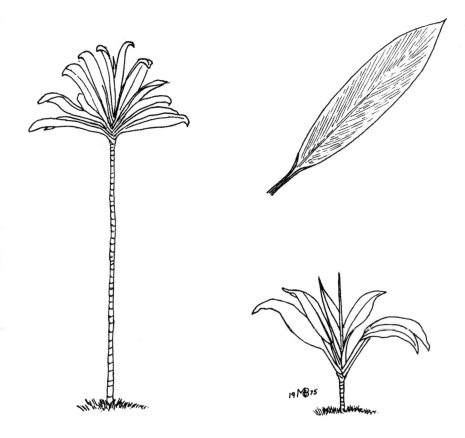

UHALOA

Waltheria americana

Uhaloa is a grayish shrub with a woody base that commonly is found inhabiting the arid sections of all of the islands at lower elevations. This perennial grows one to three feet high and has opposite leaves one to four inches long. The entire plant is covered with down and the leaves in particular are velvety and soft. The leaves are oblong ovals with a toothed margin and have conspicuous veins which are indented on the surface and correspondingly raised below. Dense clusters of tiny yellow flowers are producd on a short stalk which rises from the juncture of the leaf and the plant stem.

Both the leaves and the root of *uhaloa* are used in medicine.

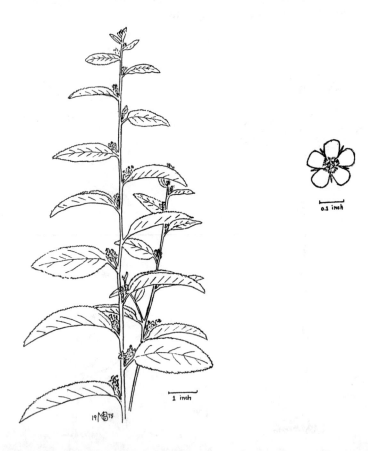

0.1 inch

1 inch

'ULEI

Osteomeles anthyllidifolia

'Ulei is a shrub with long trailing branches that in ideal conditions may grow to become a small tree. Generally, it seldom rises more than four feet from the ground and its branches arch to touch the earth up to five feet from the woody base. The brownish branches support compound leaves made up of four to nine pairs of leaflets and a terminal leaflet. On young shoots the compound leaves are arranged in a spiral up the branch which may be inconspicuous in older plants. The shiny, dark green leaflets are lighter underneath and range from one-half to three-fourths inch long. The white, five-petaled flowers which are about one-half inch in diameter give way to round, white fruits with five seeds.

'Ulei is found in the dryer open forest from sea level to about 4,000 feet altitude. The leaves and root are gathered for medicine.

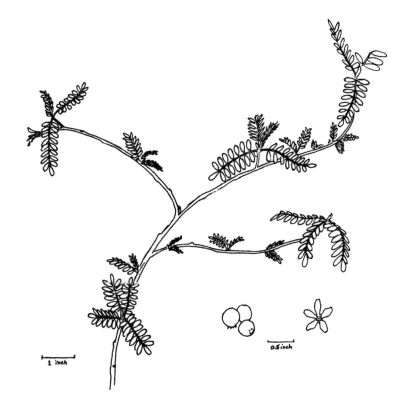

0.5 inch

1 inch

ULU

Artocarpus communis

Ulu is one of the more beautiful trees in Hawaii. It may grow to 60 feet or more in height with a diameter of about two feet. This tree is characterized by its smooth gray bark and luxuriant foliage of large, fairly dark green, deeply-lobed leaves. The large starchy fruits produced by *ulu* give the tree its common name of breadfruit.

The leathery leaves of the *ulu* tree are one to two feet long and are reminiscent of huge oak leaves. The fruit ranges in size from four to eight inches in diameter and is yellowish or brownish when ripe.

The breadfruit tree thrives in the hot wet sections of all of the islands. The milky sap is used fresh as medicine.

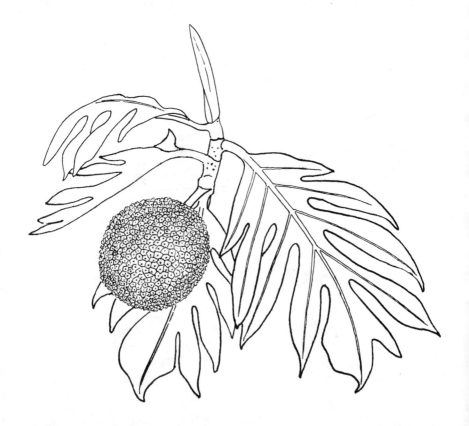

WAWAE'IOLE

Lycopodium cernuum

Wawae'iole is an extremely primitive plant found in some clearings and along the edges of woods in the uplands where the rainfall is moderate to heavy. It may grow over five feet tall in ideal situations but generally is about half that high.

The erect stem and branches are covered with tiny, pointed, scale-like leaves which give the plant a resemblance to some of the pines. The branches may fork successively, drooping in a graceful arc, terminating in a scaled green spike up to an inch long. These pendant ends produce a yellow dust that resembles pollen, but is in fact the spores by which the plant reproduces.

Wawae'iole is an evergreen with some creeping stems that root at intervals and send up new shoots. The plant is often gathered for use in flower arrangements and for decoration during Christmas time.

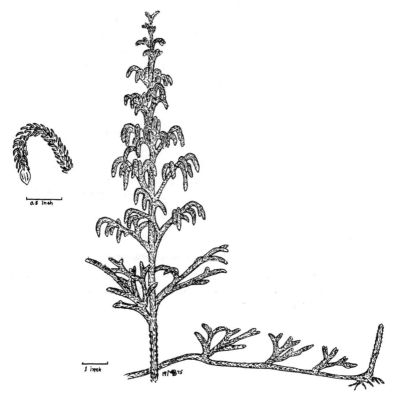

AILMENTS COMMONLY TREATED
IN HAWAIIAN FOLK MEDICINE

Appetite, Loss of
Arthritis
Asthma
Athlete's Foot

Backache
Bad Breath
Blisters
Blotchy Skin
Boils
Broken Bones
Burns

Chapped Lips
Chapped Skin
Charley Horse
Colds
Cold Hands
Cuts

Diabetes
Diarrhea
Dry Mouth

Earache
Emetic, Need of
Enema, Need of
Eyes (Weakness)

Fever
Fever Blisters
Fish Spine Wounds

Gargle, Need of
Gums, Sore

Headache
Heart Trouble
Heartburn
High Blood Pressure

Impotency
Indigestion
Infection
Inhaler, Need of
Insomnia
Kidney and Bladder
    Ailments

Laxative, Need of

Nervousness
Nettle Stings
Neuralgia

Pain
Portuguese Man-of-
    war Stings

Puncture wounds

Rash
Rheumatism

Scars
Scratches
Shock
Sinus Trouble
Skin Ailments
Sore Throat
Sprains
Stings
Stroke, Prevention
Sunburn

Tiredness
Tonic
Toothache

Wana Wounds
Warts
Wetting the Bed

Treatments are listed in alphabetical order on the following pages. In some cases there is only a reference to a statement made in the section on plant descriptions.

CAUTION: The treatments listed in this section are here only because they are a part of traditional folk medicine. Use cautiously and except in minor problems, in consultation with your doctor. These remedies have not had scientific testing.

APPETITE, LOSS OF   Refer to *Ko'oko'olau*

ARTHRITIS

Mash or grind a large fresh root of *koali* with about half as much Hawaiian salt. Spread the paste on a bandage or compress large enough to cover the afflicted area. This poultice may stain the clothes, so use caution in the application. If the fingers are to be treated, the *koali* paste can be put in an old glove, taking care to work the paste around the sore joints. The remedy should be left on for less than an hour and then sponged off gently in water as warm as the patient can stand comfortably. The area should then be kept warm and covered.

The tea to use with this treatment is made from the dried leaves of *uhaloa*. The leaves are gathered green and dried in the shade or a moderately shady place under hot, arid conditions. An alternative is to dry the leaves by placing them on a screen in an oven barely warm for several hours. A handful of dried leaves should be added to a pint of water in a pan. Bring the water to a boil and then remove the pan from the heat, cover and let the leaves steep until the tea is cool enough to drink. These remedies should be used two or three times a day for five days, and then repeated whenever necessary.   *(see 1992 Notes on page 101)*

ASTHMA

Remove the bark from an *uhaloa* root, a *popolo* root and an *olapa* root. Pound or grind these together with a piece of young *koa* bark, about four inches long by one inch. Split a joint of *ko* and grind it into the mixture. Mash one small *noni* fruit and stir it in. When all ingredients are thoroughly mixed, squeeze out the juice and strain it. A tablespoonful should be taken each morning for five days, followed by a tea made from *amaumau*.

Amaumau tea is made from the dried pith of the fern, ground to a powder. About a teaspoonful of the powder is put into a pan containing two cups of water. This should be brought to a boil and stirred well. Remove the pan from the heat and let the tea cool. Then strain it through a cloth and drink while it is still warm.

The sun-dried leaves of *puapilipili* are used for the treatment of asthma. The leaves are crushed in the hands to granulate them and then smoked in a pipe several times a day. In the same manner, the tips from *a'ali'i* branches may be dried and smoked. This treatment should not be used too often for asthma because it tends to make some patients mildly intoxicated. Chewing the fresh sticky tips of *a'ali'i* as a medication for asthma may produce much the same effect.

ATHLETE'S FOOT   Refer to BURNS

BACKACHE

Take an entire *puakala* plant and pound it with a large handful of fresh *iniko* leaves (about one cup) and a teaspoon of Hawaiian salt. You may prefer to grind the plants and then mash them with the salt in a mortar. Put the results of your work in the center of a folded towel and roll the towel lengthwise. Hold the towel over a large bowl or pan and twist the ends to put pressure on the material in the center and express the juice. To each tablespoon of this fluid add one cup of water.

Drink a small glassful of this each morning for five days. A small piece of coconut may be chewed following the drink if it is found to be somewhat disagreeable. The patient must abstain from all alcoholic beverages and coffee during the five-day treatment. Weak tea may be substituted if used in moderation.

Severe backache may be relieved by a poultice of crushed *koali* root, pounded with salt as mentioned in the treatment for arthritis. The poultice is covered with a bandage and left on for half an hour

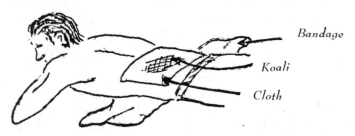

Bandage

Koali

Cloth

Backache may also result from kidney problems. See page 93.

or so while the patient is awake.

For some people a cold tea made from ripe *noni* fruit may be beneficial. The juice is squeezed from the fruit and strained through a cloth. About one tablespoon of the juice is added to a glass of water and taken several times a day.

A warm brew made from *lapine* leaves is particularly good for some kinds of backache. This tea has a pleasant citrus taste and a gingery smell. Select two or three dried leaves and wrinkle them in the hands. Then fold them in a convenient size and tie them, using one of the leaves as a cord. Drop them into boiling water, remove from heat and cover. This tea may be taken as needed each morning.

In gathering the leaves of *iniko* it is wise to use gloves to avoid the nettles on the plants.

To relieve the sting resulting from contact with *iniko* or some kinds of sugar cane, obtain a stalk of *'ape* and apply the juice of the plant to the afflicted areas.

BAD BREATH

When the teeth are clean and sound, a bad breath may be caused by sinus trouble, a coating on the tongue or an upset stomach. The *hapu'u* fern is very effective in eliminating the odor caused by the last two. Choose a frond with a downy covering on the stem that will rub off easily. The green portion thus exposed is scraped off with a knife and mashed with a pinch of Hawaiian salt. The extract is then strained through a cloth. If the bad breath is thought to originate in the mouth about a tablespoon of the juice is used as a mouthwash, swishing it around the teeth and tongue. If the bad breath is thought to be related to the stomach, the same amount of juice is swallowed. This should immediately bring up the contents of stomach. With some people it may be necessary to tickle the back of the throat with a finger to help the process. Following the emetic, a little *poi*, thinned with water, may be drunk to settle the stomach.

Bad breath caused by sinus trouble can best be dealt with by treating that affliction, followed by a gargle and the *hapu'u* mouthwash.

It is important to follow any treatment for bad breath with a thorough cleaning of the system. The patient should drink *ko'oko-'olau* tea regularly and take an effective laxative. Care should be taken not to eat too much and in particular to avoid acid foods and fresh fruits for several days.

BLISTERS

Regardless of the cause, blisters can be effectively treated by the use of *aloe* as described under the remedy for burns. If *aloe* is not available when needed, other methods of medication may be necessary.

Blisters on the hands or feet can be helped with a poultice of *popolo* leaves, mashed with a tablespoon of Hawaiian salt to make a paste. Cover the blister with the mixture and bind it in place. Sunburn blisters and blister sores on the body can be treated with a wash of vinegar several times a day. Burns can be soothed with mashed *'ape* root, mixed with juice from the stem.

BLOTCHY SKIN

According to D. M. Kaaiakamanu and J. K. Akina in *Hawaiian Herbs of Medicinal Value,* this ailment was relieved in the following manner:

"For bad blotches on the skin the meat of fresh green fruit is found most effective. To prepare it, take the meat of two young gourds *(ipu awa'awa),* the size of a large *Morinda citrifolia (noni)* fruit, and put it into about a quart of water. After being thoroughly mixed, the water from the mixture is strained and used for internal cleaning. In making the application, the water is allowed to enter the bowels slowly, the patient lying on one side and then on the other, with the region about the navel being gently shaken to allow complete distribution of the water in the intestines, thus aiding in the complete removal of all impurities from within the digestive system. For food, the patient should take roast *taro* leaves and *kukui* nut together with sweet potato."

BOILS

The most common treatment for boils is at the same time the simplest and easiest. Wash one or two moderately sized leaves of *laukahi* and take off the stems. Put a pinch or two of Hawaiian salt on a flat board and place the leaves on top. Then with a rolling pin or a bottle roll the leaves with pressure until the salt is mashed into the leaves and no lumps remain. Place the crushed *laukahi* over the boil and bandage it just firm enough to hold the poultice in place. Warm clothes held to the outside of the bandage may hasten the boil coming to a head. For a blind boil, heat the leaves thoroughly in a frying pan and bind them in place.

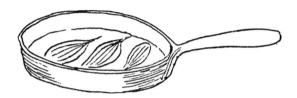

Another method of bringing a boil to a head consists of using a tablespoon of thick *poi*. Grind to dust a thumb-sized piece of the dried pith of the *amaumau* fern. Mix the *amaumau* dust thoroughly with the *poi* and then add some juice from a ripe *noni* fruit, a little at a time, until an easily spread paste is formed. Smear this paste around the boil, leaving the top exposed and warm the paste in the sun until it dries.

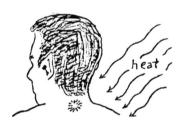

The young fronds of the *ho'i'o* fern are used in a similar fashion in treating boils. The completely dried *ho'i'o* fern shoot is ground into a dust and mixed with the milky juice from the hull of a green *kukui* nut, making a mixture that is easily spread. The paste is applied around the swelling, leaving the top uncovered, and permitted to dry in the sunshine to bring pressure on the boil and cause to burst.

BROKEN BONES

If at all possible, any broken bone should have the expert care of an attending physician. If none is available, however, the bone should be adjusted to its proper position by someone who knows the art. When the bone has been set and immobilized by splints or a sling, the healing process can begin.

Take a *koali* vine with the whole root and mash it with a handful of Hawaiian salt. If the skin has been broken, use a piece of *koa* bark about the size of the palm of the hand and two *noni* leaves and pound them all together thoroughly. Put the crushed material on the injury and bind it gently in place with a clean cloth. This treatment should be repeated every day for four days and the broken bone kept warm and still until the healing has a good start.

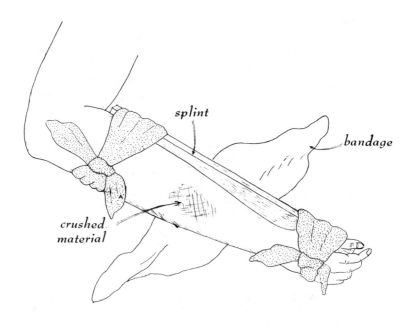

Not to be used with a plaster cast

BURNS

Several foreign plants were instantly adopted by the Hawaiians for use in medicine. One of these was the true *aloe*, whose sticky sap is taken from a fresh cut leaf and smeared gently on a burn. The injury is left uncovered unless it is very severe. Claims for the use of *aloe* on burns range from mild to miraculous. Within a generation or two, its use almost totally supplanted the former employment of 'ape root.

Aloe is also efficacious in the treatment of blisters, regardless of the cause, and is used in other remedies as well. In *Gardens of Hawaii*, Marie Neal states, "On Maui, about twenty acres of aloes have been planted since 1932, from stock long in Hawaii, to provide medicine which is used to treat athlete's foot and arthritis, when fresh to heal burns. When the leaves are cut, a thick bitter latex is drained off, which darkens and solidifies into the medicinal product."

CHAPPED LIPS

Like many other ailments, the prevention of this difficulty is easier than the cure. A tiny drop of *hinu honu* will obviate chapped lips, if applied in time. In an emergency, the oil from the side of the nose and between the chin and the lip can be rubbed on the lips with the forefinger to keep them from becoming cracked and sore. If the chapping becomes a problem, the sap from *kukui* twigs, applied to the lips, will bring relief and help to heal them.

CHAPPED SKIN

When the skin is cracked and scaly from exposure to the wind, the sap from the *ulu* tree will bring relief. Spread the fresh fluid from a cut in the bark onto the afflicted areas.

For raw places caused by excess sweating, where there is skin rubbing, *hinu honu* is especially good. Apply the oil evenly in a thin coat over the tender places. This will not only heal the injury and ease the discomfort, but will also prevent chapping if applied in time. *Hinu honu* is also excellent for the tender area that develops around the nostrils during a cold. Rub a drop of the oil around the nostrils before the nose cold becomes severe and then continue the practice until the cold ends.

CHARLEY HORSE (Cramp in leg or arm muscles)

A rounded stone four or five inches in diameter taken from a stream bed near the seacoast is a good thing to keep on hand. The use of such a stone or an iron ball, heated just hot enough, is very beneficial for the painful muscle cramp in the arm or leg, caused by overexertion. The warm ball is rolled the length of the muscle time and again, while the patient relaxes. A poultice made of *koali* root, pounded with salt, may be applied and bandaged into place to heal the damaged tissue deep inside.

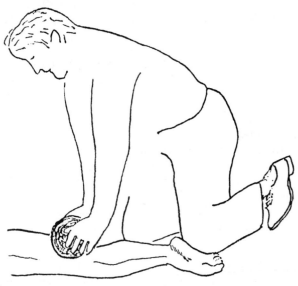

COLDS

There are probably as many remedies for the common cold in Hawaii as there are families. Many of these seem to be variations of treatments and others seem to have been imported with the ingredients they employ. The use of a tonic in treating a cold may be universal and Hawaii is no exception. The following one is simple to make and uses constituents that can be easily obtained. Soak one and one-half cups of ground *awa* root overnight in two cup of water. The following day mash together about one-fourth of a roasted *kukui* nut with ten *popolo* leaves and five tips from *ko'oko'olau* branches. Add about a teaspoon of sugar cane juice to the crushed material and mix well. Add this to the *awa* root water and stir. Strain the fluid first through a sieve and then through a cloth. Take about a tablespoon of this medicine before each meal until all of it is gone.

The person that has a cold should not neglect eating regularly, even though there might be a loss of appetite. A bundle of *popolo* leaves wrapped in *ti* leaves and steamed is said to benefit some who suffer from a cold. Select about one-half pound of young *popolo* leaves to cook at one time. The *ti* leaves are discarded and the *popolo* is divided into five parts so that one portion may be eaten with the evening meal for five days. At the end of this period a laxative should be taken to clean out the system.

A good tea to use during a cold is made from *ko'oko'olau* leaves. Bring a small pan of water to a boil and add a handful of the dried leaves. Add to this about one-quarter teaspoon of powdered *puapilipili* leaves and let the whole steep until it is cool enough to drink. The amount of *ko'oko'olau* leaves to use will vary with individual taste. This tea may be taken as frequently as desired until the cold has ended.

Palepiwa steam is good treatment for obstructed nostrils or a chest cold. Bruise a large handful of *palepiwa* leaves and put them in a pot of boiling water. Remove the pot from the fire and set it on the floor. Cover the head and shoulders with a blanket and lean over the pot, allowing the steam to rise around the head and chest. Such a steam treatment just before bedtime will help the patient sleep better.

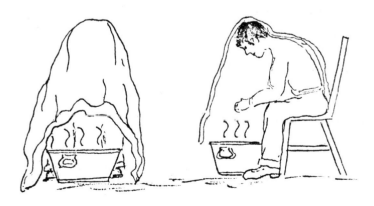

COLD HANDS

White fingertips and blotchy skin on the hands, caused by cool weather, may respond to the use of *pohe kula*. Take about a quart of the leaves and pound them together with the bark from a taproot and a tablespoon of Hawaiian salt. Put this mixture into a cloth and squeeze out the juice. Drink a teaspoonful of the juice stirred into half a glass of water, each day until it is gone. Thereafter, eat a few of the leaves every day as a salad with a meal.

CUTS

The annoying small cuts obtained during shaving can be easily treated by dipping a small *taro* stem into *noni* juice and touching it to the places. Put a small pinch of *amaumau* powder on the injury while it is still wet. This will stop the bleeding and help heal the injury.

The following recipes are for medicines used for cuts of increasing severity. For cuts that are not too deep take a double handful of leaves of *'ulei* and the bark from the root of the same plant and pound them together with a handful of Hawaiian salt. Put the result into a clean cloth and squeeze the juice into the cut. Do not bandage the injury unless it is necessary to keep it from bleeding.

Cuts from a fall and puncture wounds can be treated with an application of *koa* leaves and bark. About twenty leaves and a piece of bark about the size of a hand are pounded together with a cup of Hawaiian salt. The juice is squeezed into the cuts. Open the cloth used to express the juice and put the paste that remains against the wound, using the same cloth to bandage it if possible.

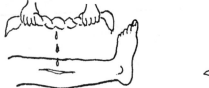 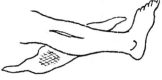

For a severe cut, pound together five leaves from sprouted coconuts with a cup of *auhuhu* leaves, a cup of *kuawa* buds, about two tablespoons of *ha'uoi* flowers and buds and a cup of Hawaiian salt. Squeeze the juice directly into the cut from a clean cloth. This treatment is quite painful and it might be wise to have a strong person hold the patient while another administers the remedy.

DIABETES   Refer to *Noni*

DIARRHEA

When the bowels are too loose from the onset of a cold, having eaten something disagreeable or having overdosed with a laxative, *pia* will arrest the difficulty. Put a tablespoonful of *pia* starch into a small amount of previously mixed *poi*. Make sure that it is mixed well and that all the lumps are out. Then add *poi* to taste and eat the entire amount.

Pia starch may be purchased at health food stores on most of the islands. If desired, you can make your own starch by grating fresh *pia*. The arrowroot tubers are first peeled and then finely grated in water. The water is then decanted and the starch washed many times with fresh water. Letting it soak and agitating it periodically will help it sweeten more quickly. Dry the starch on muslin or thin sailcloth in the sun.

Eating Kuawa buds is also an effective remedy for diarrhea

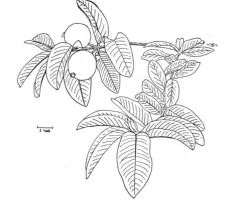

DRY MOUTH

The root of *ilie'e* is a rapid remedy for those who suffer from a dry mouth caused by fear or excitement. Peel a piece of the root about as large as the first joint of the little finger. Crush the root between the teeth and shift the material around in the mouth.

Although *ilie'e* is said by some to be poisonous, the small amount of juice that is swallowed during this treatment has never proved harmful. The patient should spit out all of the root fiber and rinse the mouth once with a little fresh water.

EARACHE

Cut the section between the leaves and the root from two very young *ti* plants. Remove the outer bark and grind them with a pinch of Hawaiian salt. Peel a medium-sized bulb of *aka'akai* and grind it into the same container. Mix the juices and strain them into a pan and place the pan in hot water in order to heat the juices. Have the patient put his head on the side with the sore ear up. Test the temperature of the medicine on the wrist and, using a teaspoon, drop it into the ailing ear. After some minutes permit the ear to drain and let the patient hold a very warm rock wrapped in a towel on the afflicted ear. This treatment should be repeated several times a day for five days.

EMETIC, NEED OF

When there is reason to cause vomiting to clean out the system, *ti* leaves are very beneficial. Scrape the dark green side of the leaves with a knife to obtain a handful of the material. Put the scrapings into about two cups of fresh water. Buy a fairly fresh *uwala* (sweet-potato), about the size of two fingers, and grind it into the water with the *ti* scrapings. Stir this together and strain it through a cloth. Drink as much of the fluid as possible and put the finger down the throat to start the process. A drink of cool fresh water will stop the vomiting.

ENEMA, NEED OF

A powerful enema is made from fresh *kukui* nuts and water. Two green *kukui* nuts are mashed and mixed with about a quart of fresh water. The mixture is then strained through a cloth and administered to the patient who lies on the stomach with a pad or cushion under the abdomen. The patient then rolls slowly on one side and then the other until the fluid can no longer be contained.

Another enema is described under the treatment for blotchy skin.

EYES (Weakness)

The dry yellow husks of *aka'akai* are said to be good for the eyes. A handful of the clean husks are boiled in a small pan of water and permitted to cool. The husks are removed from the water and the fluid drunk as a tea a little bit every day to give strength to the eyes.

FEVER

Since the introduction of aspirin into Hawaii not many of the old remedies are used to reduce fever. If this modern method is unavailable or the patient cannot use aspirin, a recourse is to employ an older method.

Have the patient, divested of clothing, lie on a bed or *pune'e.* Cover the entire body with large *ti* leaves from the neck to the feet, overlapping the leaves to make a kind of sweat bath to help break the fever. Fresh water may be given in small amounts from time to time, if the sufferer is conscious. After several hours the patient will begin to sweat, showing that the fever has broken. Remove the *ti* leaves and keep the patient warm.

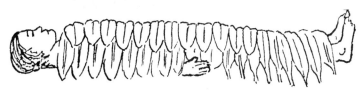

A similar treatment consists of covering a mat with *koa* leaves and having the patient lie on them. The person being treated should be well covered with a blanket and periodically given *ko'oko'olau* tea to drink. After the fever victim has begun to sweat and the fever is broken, remove the *koa* leaves and keep the patient warm and quiet.

A kind of a sponge bath using *oliwa-ku-kahakai* will give immediate relief to a person with a fever. Crush about a quart of the leaves with a tablespoon of Hawaiian salt and put the result into a cheese cloth. Gently wipe the torso and limbs with the saturated cloth with special attention to the back of the neck and underarms. When sponging the face be careful not to get any of the juice into the eyes.

FEVER BLISTER

Burn to ashes several fronds of *pi'ipi'i-lau-manamana*. To about a tablespoon of the fern ashes, add enough to the fresh sap of *ulu* to make a paste. Daub the blister with the paste and let it dry. Continue the treatment until the blister forms a scab.

Another remedy employs the use of the green moss *iliole*. The sun-dried moss is pounded to a powder. Mash two young green *kukui* nuts with a little Hawaiian salt and squeeze out the juice into a small container. Add enough of the *iliohe* dust to make a paste and apply it to the blister.

Some fever blisters respond to the remedy using *limu-kaha*. Thoroughly mash a handful of the *limu-kaha* and strain it through a cloth. Add the juice to about half a cup of *okolehao*, a liquor distilled from *ti root*. Saturate a piece of cotton or *pulu* and daub the blister frequently with the mixture.

The sticky sap from *aloe* smeared on a fever blister is said by some to be efficacious.

FISH SPINE WOUNDS   Refer to STINGS

GARGLE, NEED OF

When the *kukui* trees are in bloom is the time to make a good gargle. Gather about a quart of the blossoms and a piece of the *kukui* bark about the size of a hand. Obtain a piece of *ohia-lehua* bark the same size from a young tree. Grind or pound all of these together with a tablespoon of Hawaiian salt and strain the mixture through a cloth. Add to the mixture the milk from a ripe coconut. This may be refrigerated and used when necessary.

About a tablespoon of Hawaiian salt dissolved in a pint of fresh water also makes a good gargle.

GUMS, SORE

Sore gums may respond to the use of the water from a green coconut. The fluid is drained from the unripe fruit and rubbed on the gums with the finger. Following this application, drink one-half cup of the coconut water three times a day for five days.

HEADACHE

Awa is very good for migraine and the headache that comes with tension. Put a few small pieces of the root in the mouth at a time and chew them. Add a few more pieces until a cud or bolus about the size of the thumb is formed. Three of these lumps of chewed *awa* root are sufficient to make a drink that is a remedy for headache. Put the awa cuds into a bowl and mash them with about a cup of fresh water. Strain the fluid through a cloth to remove the woody material and drink the liquid. A weaker drink can be made by grinding the *awa* root instead of chewing it. If the medicine is too bitter, eat a few *pupu* to remove the taste.

For the ache that comes with a bump on the head take four roots of *awapuhi* the size of a man's thumb and pound them with about a tablespoon of Hawaiian salt. Dip a cloth into the juice and apply to the head around and on the injury.

Green *ti* leaves held at the temples and the forehead are helpful in relieving some kinds of headache.

HEART TROUBLE   Refer to *Noni*

HEARTBURN

Take four young shoots of *pakikawaio* and grind them with a quart of fresh *iliohe*. Mash this with two tablespoons of Hawaiian salt and add a dozen well cooked young taro leaves. Let this be the only food for a day and *koʻokoʻolau* tea and fresh water the only fluids. The following day take a mild laxative and eat sparingly. Tobacco and alcohol should be avoided during the treatment.

HIGH BLOOD PRESSURE

A mild tea of koʻokoʻolau taken 4 times a day for 5 days, then none for 2 days as long as necessary.   *(see 1992 Notes on page 101)*

IMPOTENCY

Remove the bark from four *olapa* roots and pound them with an equal amount of *pipi* and two joints of *ko*. Add a quart of fresh water, mix and strain through a cloth. Drink half a cup of this fluid morning and evening until it is gone. Tobacco and alcohol should be avoided during the treatment.

INDIGESTION

Break off a piece of *awapuhi pake* about the size of two joints of a finger. Put this root in a pan containing a quart of fresh water and bring it to a boil and let it simmer for a few minutes. Cool the tea and drink about a cupful before each meal until the malady is relieved.

INFECTION

If possible open the wound and permit it to drain. Pound a hand-sized piece of the inner bark of *koa* with two tablespoons of Hawaiian salt. Allow the *koa* juice to drip into the injury and plaster the fiber against the infection and bind it on with a cloth. Repeat the treatment morning and evening, leaving the wound open to the sunlight in the warm afternoon.

Some infections will respond to the use of *taro* leaves. Mash six medium-sized *taro* leaves with a handful of Hawaiian salt. Apply this poultice to the injury and cover it with a large *taro* leaf. If the infection is on a limb, wrap the leaf around and bandage it in place. The poultice should be changed three times a day until the infection is gone.

INHALER, NEED OF

Mash a pint of the tender tips of *a'ali'i* with ten flowers of *awapuhi keokeo*. Express about a tablespoon of juice from a joint of *ko* and combine it with the *a'ali'i* and the blossoms. Add a ball of *pulu* about the size of a man's thumb and mix all together well. Allow the mixture to dry in the sun until it can be rolled into sicks smaller than the little finger. When these are dry enough to hold together they are ready to use in the nostril.

This inhaler is said to improve the disposition and clear the head of those who use it. It is also helpful for shortness of breath.

INSOMNIA

For mild sleeplessness gather the sticky tips of the *a'ali'i* bushes. These are dried slowly under hot shaded conditions. They may be stored in an airtight container and used as tobacco. Two or three pipefuls, when one is wakeful, should be enough to cause drowsiness.

The use of *awa* to induce sleep is thousands of years old. Prepare the *awa root* as recommended in the remedy for headache. If a sufficient quantity is consumed, the patient will enjoy many hours of refreshing sleep without feeling "hung over" when awakened. According to D. M. Kaaiakamanu and J. K. Akina in *Hawaiian Herbs of Medicinal Value,* severe insomnia was treated with *ipu awaawa*. Its young shoot and the leaves close to it are very helpful in case of partial insanity due to lack of sleep. The patient takes these and eats them. This is followed by the chewing of a piece of dried coconut with sweet potato and a drink of water. This is done twice a day for five successive times. After the treatments, a whole day of rest is taken, after which the patient, using the meat or scraping from the inside of two fully matured or thoroughly ripe fruits, takes an internal bath to clean out his bowels and, with about a quart of water, he is given an external bath.

KIDNEY and BLADDER AILMENTS

Express the juice from a quart of *ohelo kau la'au* berries, using a sturdy piece of denim. Remove the skins and seeds from the cloth and crush them in a mortar. Add the mashed seeds and skins to the juice and let the mixture stand for several hours. Strain the juice through a cloth that will take out the seeds and refrigerate it. Take a tablespoonful of the juice before each meal and before bedtime for five days. Drink plenty of fluids but avoid alcohol and coffee. You may substitute cranberry juice, but double the amount taken.

LAXATIVE

The following internal cleansing agents are listed in the order that they are easiest to secure. A few leaves of *laukahi* chewed and swallowed are a mild laxative for most people, with an added advantage of little work involved in preparing it.

In some places *hau* flowers are common and require no labor to use as a laxative. The base of the flower is chewed and swallowed. It is best to start with a few to see what your own tolerance is.

The easiest natural laxative to keep on hand is *kukui*. The mature *kukui* nuts are gathered and the shells cracked by putting them in a vise and exerting pressure slowly. The nut meat is removed from the shell and roasted in a medium oven for an hour. If each nut meat is folded in a piece of aluminum foil before roast-

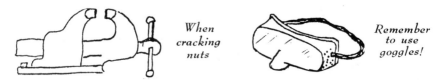

When cracking nuts

Remember to use goggles!

ing, it can be kept and stored in this package for future use. Try a pinch or so of the roasted *kukui* to determine its effect on you. This is a powerful purge so exercise caution in the amount you take and keep the *kukui* nuts away from children.

For those who are concerned with regularity one-fourth cup of sea water obtained from a clean source can be taken every morning after arising.

If any laxative has too much effect, this can be stopped by taking a tablespoon of *pia* starch in a glass of water.

NERVOUSNESS

Awa prepared as directed for headache, is also good for a nervous condition. This should not be taken too often or in too great a quantity because of certain undesirable side effects. Abuse of this drug will cause the skin to scale and peel as with sunburn. The flaking is especially noticeable at the elbows, knees and the back of the neck.

Lomi (massage) is especially good for nervousness when practiced by a master of this Hawaiian art. Some claim to have been cured of this ailment by the manipulation of the muscles and bones. If an expert is unavailable, a simple rub-down and massage are helpful in treating the patient.

NETTLE STINGS   Refer to BACKACHE

NEURALGIA

Grind the bark of four *uhaloa* roots and two handfuls of *awa*. Put this in a pan with six cups of cold water and bring to a boil. Reduce the heat and let the brew simmer for about ten to fifteen minutes with a cover on it. Remove the pan from the heat and when cool, strain the mixture through a cloth. Drink one-half cup of this tea twice a day for five days. If the taste is disagreeable eat a small banana or a piece of dried coconut. A laxative should be taken at the completion of the treatment.

PAIN

When injuries or other conditions cause pain, it can be relieved by the mixture of several plants. Clean two entire *puakala* and grind or pound them with four *pipi*, the bark from six *uhaloa* roots, and a quart of the small leaves and buds of *uhaloa*. Add a tablespoon of Hawaiian salt and mix thoroughly. Let the mixture stand for a few minutes. Add a pint of fresh water, stir and strain through a cloth. Squeeze the cloth well to get all of the juice out. Put the fluid into a glass jar and refrigerate it until it is needed. Shake the jar to stir up the dregs before using. Take a tablespoonful every few hours as long as the pain persists. Follow the treatment with a laxative.

For occasional chest pain crush a ripe *noni* fruit and strain the juice into a quart of water. Add a tablespoon of this to a glass of prepared *awa* drink as described for headache.

PORTUGUESE MAN-OF-WAR STINGS
Refer to STINGS

PUNCTURE WOUNDS

The various treatments for puncture wounds that have been selected derive their main ingredients from different locations on the islands. For such an injury at the beach, remove the bark from a root of *naupaka kahakai* and pound it with a handful of Hawaiian salt. Squeeze out the juice into puncture, working it as deep as possible with the fingers. From the same plant get a handful of leaves and mash them with a little salt and apply this as a poultice and bind it over the wound.

In the mountains, such an injury can be treated with an application of *koa* leaves and bark. About 20 leaves and a hand-sized piece of young *koa* bark are pounded together with a cup of Hawaiian salt. The juice is expressed into the wound. The fiber mass is then put over the puncture and bandaged in place.

At the intermediate altitudes the remedy for puncture wounds uses two plants that are common there. Pound or grind an entire *koali* vine and root with four young shoots of *kuawa* and a cup of Hawaiian salt. Squeeze the juice of these into the injury and work it as deep inside as possible. Bandage some of the material against the wound. This may be repeated twice a day until healing begins.

RASH

This ailment is best treated internally and externally at the same time. The bath or wash should not be neglected. To prepare it, collect about 40 *auhuhu* leaves, four pieces of *puakala* root bark, and a quart of *a'ali'i* leaves. Pound all of these together with a teaspoon of Hawaiian salt. Strain the mixture through a cloth and add it to a gallon of fresh water in a pan. Bring the solution to a boil, cover it and let it simmer over reduced heat for half an hour. When the bath is cool enough, sponge the body with the solution. Do this several times a day until the rash and its itching go away.

The internal treatment consists of a glass of *awa* prepared by the method outlined for a headache. Drink this much twice a day as long as the bath treatment lasts.

RHEUMATISM

Formerly the Hawaiians were said to treat rheumatism with a bath made by boiling *wawaeiole,* a lycopod found in the wet areas of the mountains. Remedies involving the use of imported trees seem to be more popular today.

Bruise about two quarts of *palepiwa* leaves and a small piece of

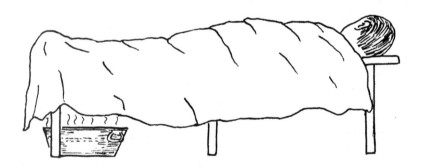

A WOODEN COT IS EXCELLENT FOR THIS REMEDY.   ADDITIONAL BOILING WATER MAY BE USED TO PROLONG THE TREATMENT.

the bark. Boil these in a gallon or two of water for an hour. Bathe the sore joints with the warm solution. Dry hot cloths held to the afflicted area will be useful at night.

Another method of treating rheumatism consists of several parts. Pound or grind about a quart of *pepa* leaves and put the result into a gallon of water. Bring it to a boil and simmer it for several minutes. Drape the patient in a blanket to make a tent over the body but with the head outside. Put the steaming container underneath, near the patient's feet. Allow the steam to envelope the entire body. When the solution is cool enough, sponge the sore joints. This is done morning and evening for five days. In between the baths the afflicted should absorb as much sun on the body as tolerable. Keep the patient warm and comfortable at all times. Give *ko'oko'olau* tea to drink several times a day for the duration of the medication. At that time administer a laxative to clean out the system.

SCARS

After a cut has closed and the healing process has begun, massage the surface gently with *hinu honu* several times a day. This will make the scar as small as possible and perhaps eliminate it entirely.

Aloe is said to be beneficial as well in reducing scar tissue. The gelatinous interior of the leaf is applied two or three times a day.

SCRATCHES

Most scratches can be treated with a little salt crushed as fine as possible and sprinkled on the area. The milky sap of *ulu* applied directly to the scratch will prevent inflammation and start the healing.

SHOCK

When a person has been badly injured, it is important to treat the victim for shock immediately. If the patient is conscious, administer a half-cup of salt water followed by a half-cup of water sweetened with *ko* juice. Half a teaspoon of each in the water will suffice.

SINUS TROUBLE

Clean sea water is one of the best medications for sinusitis. Take a little ocean water into the cup of the hand and snuff it up the nostrils. This is done five times a day for five days and thereafter only once a day to prevent a recurrence.

If the forehead and cheekbones ache from pressure in the sinus, drink an ounce of *okolehao* or other strong alcoholic beverage. Then bruise 40 leaves of *palepiwa* and bring them to a boil in a gallon of water. Hold a towel over the head and let the steam come up against the face for about 15 minutes. The patient then lies on his back while a towel saturated with the hot solution is wrung out and placed on his face. This should be continued until the patient is able to sleep. The sufferer should remain on his back without turning for the best effect. This remedy should be repeated twice a day until the sinus pressure is relieved. A gargle should be included in the final treatment, along with the remedies for sore throat and bad breath if necessary.

SKIN AILMENTS

Cracked skin, blotches, itch, scale ringworm and other disorders may be treated by the use of *ha'uoi*. Grind an entire plant with a tablespoon of Hawaiian salt and strain the juice through a cloth. Bathe the afflicted areas with the fluid and dust with *pia* starch. Repeat the process four times a day until the ailment heals. Coconut milk diluted with water may be used to clean off the medication.

Sores and ulcers are treated in a similar manner. Burn to ashes a dried frond of *pi'ipi'i-lau-manamana*. Crush two young green *kukui* nuts and apply the milk to the sore, using a small wad of *pulu*. Sprinkle the sore with the ashes. On difficult areas a paste of the *kukui* milk and ashes may be used.

In treating any skin ailments, the patient should not forget to clean out the system by drinking *ko'oko'olau* tea and taking a laxative.

SORE THROAT
The use of *uhaloa* in the treatment of sore throat is no doubt one of the best known folk remedies in Hawaii. The bark of the root is chewed and the juice permitted to coat the throat as it is swallowed. This is done several times a day until the soreness is gone.

SPRAINS
Severe sprains should be treated with the same medication as broken bones for rapid healing. Slight sprains may be helped with a combination of several plants. Grind or pound a root of *ilie'e* with an equal amount of *awapuhi* root and a ripe *noni* fruit. Put the pulp in a cloth and bind it loosely around the injured part. Change the dressing every day until the sprain has healed. Warming the injury in the afternoon sun will help promote a rapid recovery.

STINGS
A sting from a honey bee must be examined immediately to locate the stinger which generally remains in the skin. Remove it with tweezers, taking care not squeeze the poison sac on the end. Pound a *mikana* leaf and apply it as a poultice on the swelling and bind it in place. The milky juice from a green fruit can be used as an alternative if that is more available. This remedy is also good for Portuguese man-of-war stings and fish spine wounds.

STROKE, PREVENTION OF   Refer to *Ko'oko'olau*

SUNBURN
The sap of young *kukui* nuts will bring relief from mild overexposure to the sun. More severe cases can be treated with the gelatinous interior of *aloe* leaves.

Sunburn can be prevented by an application of *hinu honu* on exposed areas of the skin. Wherever this oil is rubbed, the sunlight will not penetrate. Unfortunately, it also prevents sun-tanning as well.

TIREDNESS

Awa prepared as indicated for the treatment of headache is also good for tiredness. The diet should be checked to insure that enough different kinds of food are included. Red salt may be substituted for the customary white product. If the person is already getting enough rest, a tonic followed by a laxative may be beneficial.

TONIC, NEED OF

Pound together a quart of red and pink *ohia* tips, a handful of *ihi leaves,* a thumb-sized piece of *alaea* earth and a joint of *ko.* Add a pint of fresh water and stir well. Strain the mixture through a cloth and refrigerate in a container that can be shaken. Take a tablespoon of this tonic (well shaken) in half a glass of water before each meal for five days. *Lapine* tea should be drunk two or three times a day. A laxative should be taken to cleanse the system at the end of the treatment.

TOOTHACHE

For a tooth with a cavity cook a small piece of *awapuhi* root in a frying pan to soften it. Bite down on the root to press it into the hollow and leave it there as long as necessary. If a filling has been lost and the tooth is otherwise sound, collect the sap from an *ulu* tree and let it dry into gum. Mold the bit of gum to fit the socket of the filling and press in place. The toothache may be treated as for pain and a glass or two of prepared *awa* will help the patient to sleep.

WANA WOUND

An injury caused by stepping on a *wana* or sea urchin can be treated with the patient's own urine to bring relief. If the sufferer is squeamish, vinegar may be used as a substitute.

This affliction may also respond to the treatment used for stings and punctures by fish spines.

WARTS

The application of *hinu honu* to a wart along with gentle massage several times a day will sometimes cause a wart to go away entirely.

WETTING THE BED

Awa, prepared as described for a headache, is useful for alleviating this problem. Drink a small glass of *awa* about an hour before going to bed. Remember to void the bladder before retiring.

1992 Notes

ARTHRITIS

For swollen joints of the hands two more things are recommended:

A piece of steam-cooked sweet potato five inches long and an inch in diameter eaten five times a week skin and all, alleviates the pain in some cases within a month or two. (Do not substitute yams. They belong to a different family).

Some people find relief by adding a sprinkle of hot pepper flakes, seeds and all, (the kind often found in pizza parlors) to a suitable food every day for five days until the joints are no longer painful.

HIGH BLOOD PRESSURE

It has been suggested recently that ripe noni fruit processed in a blender with water and refrigerated is helpful for this disorder. The fruit should be yellow and only slightly soft. A cup of the juice twice a day is recommended.

HAWAIIAN WORDS USED IN THE TEXT

kahakai . . . . beach, seashore
kahuna . . . . an expert in any profession
kahuna lapa'au la'au . . . . a *kahuna* specializing in healing with the use of herbs
kama'aina . . . . child of the land, old timer
kapu . . . . taboo, forbidden
loa . . . . long
lomi lomi . . . . massage
mahalo . . . . thank you
nui . . . . great, large, very much
o'o . . . . digging implement
okolehao . . . . liquor distilled from the fermented roots of *ti*
puka . . . . perforation, hole
pulu . . . . yellow, cotton-like material on the base of tree fern stems
pune'e . . . . moveable couch
pupu . . . . general name for sea and land shells, hors d'oeuvres

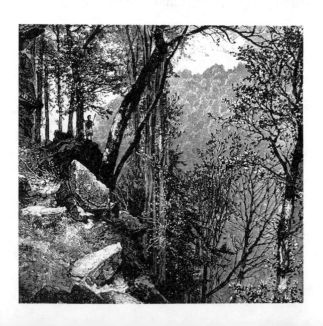

About the Author
L.R. McBride

The author and illustrator of PRACTICAL FOLK MEDICINE OF HAWAII lived at Volcano, Hawai'i for many years. He was a student of all things Hawaiian and lectured on geology, botany, history and legends of Hawai'i. His death in October 1992 has left a great void.

Of part Seneca Indian descent, Mr. McBride grew up in Ohio, where as a child he first became interested in medicinal plants. He received a B.S. degree in geology from Ohio State University, with a minor in botany. In an eleven year association with the National Park Service at Hawai'i Volcanoes National Park, Mr. McBride continued to add to his knowledge of all things Hawaiian.

The author wrote and illustrated four other outstanding original works: ABOUT HAWAII'S VOLCANOES; PETROGLYPHS OF HAWAII; THE KAHUNA, VERSATILE MYSTICS OF OLD HAWAII; and PELE, VOLCANO GODDESS OF HAWAII. He was also the illustrator of KONA LEGENDS by Eliza Maguire.

Mr. McBride was known as a botanical illustrator and is listed as such in the Twentieth Century Botanical Art and Illustration Index.

From a review in Phytologia, v. 34, page 1

Practical Folk Medicine, by L. R. McBride

"*L. Richard McBride, former Ranger of Hawaii Volcanoes National Park and presently Lecturer at Kilauea Military Camp, has authored his sixth book, 'Practical Folk Medicine of Hawaii.' This book of 104 pages is illustrated with 84 figures, over half of plants used by ancient kahunalapa'au, or medicine men. McBride, under one of his nine headings, warns the reader that his 'doctor be consulted' before using a home remedy. Hence the book is not a danger to health and even life of the gullible reader as is the disaster authored by Kaalakamana and Akina in 1922 and unfortunately recently reprinted.....'Practical Folk Medicine' caters to the resident and tourist interested in Hawaiiana and local plants in general.....it is of value to workers in pharmacology of the world as it gives them a clue as to which Hawaiian plants deserve assay. Who knows what medical discoveries the kahunalapa'au has made, and how modern chemists may improve on them to enhance their efficacy.*"

Otto and Isa Degener

BOOKS TO READ

Arnold, H. L. *Poisonous Plants of Hawaii.* 1968

Buck, Peter. *Arts and Crafts of Hawaii.* 1957
(Available as separate chapters paperbound or from the Book Gallery in a hardbound cloth edition.)

Degener, Dr. Otto. *Flora Hawaiiensis.* 1946 3 vols.

Degener, Dr. Otto. *Plants of the Hawaii National Park*

Handy, E. S. *The Hawaiian Planter.* 1940

Handy, E. S. and E. G. *Native Planters of Old Hawaii.* 1972

Handy, E. S. *Outline of Hawaiian Physical Therapeutics.* 1934

Ii, J. P. *Fragments of Hawaiian History.* 1959

Kaaiakamanu, D. M. and J. K. Akina. *Hawaiian Herbs of Medicinal Value.* 1922

Kamakau, S. M. *Ka Poe Kahiko, the People of Old.* 1964

Malo, David. *Hawaiian Antiquities.* 1951

Miller, C. D. *Food Values of Breadfruit, Taro Leaves, Coconut and Sugar Cane.* 1929

Miller, C. D. *The Fruits of Hawaii.* 1965

Moon, Jan. *Living with Nature in Hawaii.* 1971

Neal, M. C. *In Gardens of Hawaii.* 1965

Pukui, M. K. and S. H. Elbert. *Hawaiian English Dictionary.* 1974

Rotar, P. P. *Grasses of Hawaii.* 1968

Teho, Fortunato. *Plants of Hawaii and How to Grow Them.*